Histology at a Glance

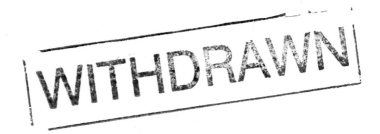

A useful website which can be used alongside this book is available at:

www.wiley.com/go/ histologyataglance

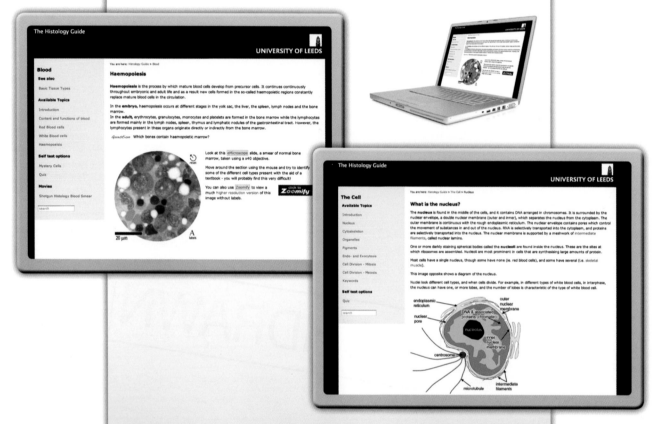

The site was developed by the author of *Histology at a Glance* and the University of Leeds.

The site includes:

- Histological slides with on/off labels for all the main body systems
- Topic objectives
- Self-test quizzes
- Histological movies

Histology
at a Glance

Michelle Peckham

BA (York), PhD (London)
Professor of Cell Biology
Institute for Molecular and Cellular Biology
Faculty of Biological Sciences
University of Leeds
Leeds, UK

WILEY-BLACKWELL

A John Wiley & Sons, Ltd., Publication

Registered office: John Wiley & Sons Ltd, The Atrium, Southern Gate, Chichester, West Sussex, PO19 8SQ, UK

Editorial offices: 9600 Garsington Road, Oxford, OX4 2DQ, UK

The Atrium, Southern Gate, Chichester, West Sussex, PO19 8SQ, UK

111 River Street, Hoboken, NJ 07030-5774, USA

For details of our global editorial offices, for customer services and for information about how to apply for permission to reuse the copyright material in this book please see our website at www.wiley.com/wiley-blackwell

Library of Congress Cataloging-in-Publication Data is available

ISBN: 978-1-4443-3332-9

A catalogue record for this book is available from the British Library.

Set in 9 on 11.5 pt Times NR MT by Toppan Best-set Premedia Limited

Printed and bound in Singapore by Markono Print Media Pte Ltd

1 2011

Contents

Companion website

A useful website which can be used alongside this book is
available at:

www.wiley.com/go/histologyataglance
The site was developed by the author of *Histology at a
Glance* and the University of Leeds.

The site includes:
- Histological slides with on/off labels for all the main body
  systems
- Topic objectives
- Self-test quizzes
- Histological movies

Preface

The aim of this book is to provide a concise overview of histology, particularly for those students who have not studied histology before. The most common complaint that I hear from students studying histology for the first time is that 'everything looks pink', which makes it difficult to understand what they are looking at.

The images used in each chapter of this book are aimed to help students to understand quickly how tissues are made up from same basic components, and how the organization and appearance of cells in each tissue varies, depending on the function of the tissue.

Acknowledgments

The author would like to thank Tim Lee, Paul Drake, Adele Knibbs, and Steve Paxton at the University of Leeds, for their advice and help in generating some of the images. She would also like to thank her family (James, Helena, Alasdair, and Gabriel) for their support, while putting the book together.

List of abbreviations

ACE	angiotensin-converting enzyme
ACTH	adrenocorticotropic hormone
ADH	antidiuretic hormone
AML	acute myeloid leukemia
A-V	atrio-ventricular
CCK	cholecystokinin
CD	cluster of differentiation markers
CLL	chronic lymphocytic leukemia
CNS	central nervous system
DCT	distal convoluted tubule
ECM	extracellular matrix
EEL	external elastic layer (of tunica media)
ER	endoplasmic reticulum
ERS	external root sheath (of hair follicle)
FAE	follicle-associated epithelial (cells)
FSH	follicle-stimulating hormone
GAG	glycosaminoglycan
GALT	gut-associated lymphoid tissue
H&E	hematoxylin & eosin
IEL	inner elastic layer (of tunica intima)
IRS	internal root sheath (of hair follicle)
LH	luteinizing hormone
MALT	mucosa-associated lymphoid tissue
NMJ	neuromuscular junction
PALS	periarteriolar lymphoid sheath
PAS	periodic acid–Schiff (reaction)
PCT	proximal convoluted tubule
PNS	peripheral nervous system
PTH	parathyroid hormone
RPE	retinal pigment epithelium
S-A	sino-atrial
SR	sarcoplasmic reticulum
T3	tri-iodothyronine
T4	thyroxine
TSH	thyroid-stimulating hormone
ZF	zona fasciculata
ZG	zona glomerulosa
ZR	zona reticularis

1 Preparation of tissues for histology

(a) Fixation

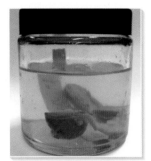

First the tissue is placed in fixative and allowed to fix

(b) Dehydration, clearing and wax impregnation

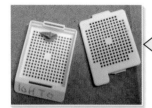

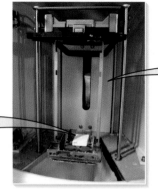

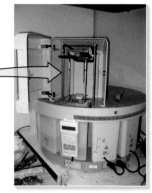

Next, the tissue is trimmed and placed in a cassette (the two halves of which are shown here)

The holder is placed in a basket in the automatic processor

The processor transfers the tissue through a series of alcohol solutions of increasing strength, and then into a clearing agent (xylene) and finally into molten wax to complete the wax impregnation process

(c) Embedding

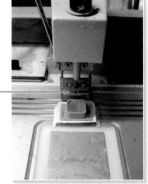

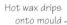

Hot wax drips onto mould

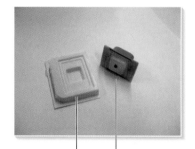

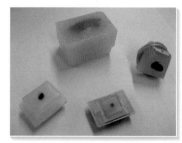

The mould   The finished block

Blocks come in all shapes and sizes, depending on the size of the tissue

The tissue is transferred to a mould, and hot wax is dispensed into the mould

(d) Sectioning

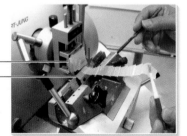

Block
Knife edge

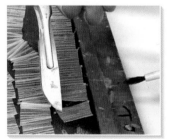

The block is moved up and down (red arrow) and moved incrementally forward (toward the user) to cut sections. Serial sections emerge in a long ribbon, and are picked up with brushes

Single sections are picked up, floated on the surface of hot water, which removes the folds, and then transferred onto a glass slide

(e) Staining

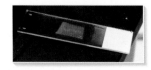

The unstained section on the slide

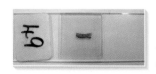

The final slide after staining and mounting

Histology is the study of tissues and their appearance.

Histos is Greek for 'web or tissue', and *logia* is Greek for 'branch of learning'.

Anatomists first used the word 'tissue' to describe the different textures of parts of the body, as they were being dissected.

Today, histology and pathology (the study of diseased tissues) are routinely used in hospitals and research laboratories to study the organization of tissues and the cells within them.

Sectioning and preparing tissue for staining

To study the structures of cells and their organization within tissues, tissues have to be fixed and 'sectioned' (or cut), stained with dyes, and then observed with the light microscope. This is carried out in the following stages (see Fig. 1).

Fixation

A chemical solution containing a fixative at pH 7.0 is added to the tissue (Fig. 1a). The most commonly used fixative is formaldehyde at a concentration of 4%. (Commonly, dilutions are made from a stock of Formalin, i.e., 37% or 40% formaldehyde.) Formaldehyde binds to and cross-links some proteins, and denatures others, but does not interact well with lipids. The overall effect is to harden the tissue and inactivate enzymes, preventing the tissue from degrading.

Dehydration

In order for sections to be cut, the tissue has to be embedded in wax. However, wax is not soluble in water. Therefore, the water in the tissue has to be removed and eventually replaced with a medium in which wax *is* soluble. This is achieved by, first, sequentially replacing the water with alcohol, placing the tissue in a series of solutions that contain increasing concentrations of alcohol, ending at 100% (Fig. 1b). This process is carried out gradually in order to minimize tissue damage. The tissue must then be 'cleared' before it can be embedded in wax.

Clearing

Next, the section is placed in an organic solvent such as xylene or toluene, which replaces the alcohol. Wax is not soluble in alcohol. The clearing agents are so-called, because the tissue often looks completely clear when it is immersed in clearing agent. Finally, the tissue is impregnated with hot wax (Fig. 1b), which is soluble in this type of organic solvent.

Embedding

The tissue is placed in warm paraffin wax in a mould (Fig. 1c). On subsequent cooling, the wax hardens, and tissue slices can now be cut.

Sectioning

Sections (slices) about 10 to 20 microns (μm) thick are cut using a microtome (Fig. 1d).

Mounting

The wax sections are laid onto a glass microscope slide (Fig. 1e).

Staining

To see detail, the components of the tissue have to be stained. However, the stains that are used are all aqueous. Therefore, the wax has to be dissolved and replaced with water (rehydration), for the stains to be able to penetrate the tissue section. The sections are therefore placed in decreasing concentrations of alcohol, ending up at 0% alcohol (water).

A number of different stains can be used but the most common is hematoxylin & eosin (see Chapter 2).

Dehydration and mounting

The stained specimen is once again dehydrated, before placing it into mounting medium dissolved in xylene. Finally, a coverslip is placed on top of the sample to protect it, and the slide can be viewed on the microscope.

Other types of sectioning

Frozen sections

The tissue is rapidly frozen, fixed, and slices cut using a cryostat, before staining.

Semi-thin sections

The tissue is embedded in epoxy or acrylic resin, which has different properties to wax, and allows thinner sections (less than 2 μm) to be cut.

Sections in electron microscopy

See Chapter 4.

2 Different types of histological stain

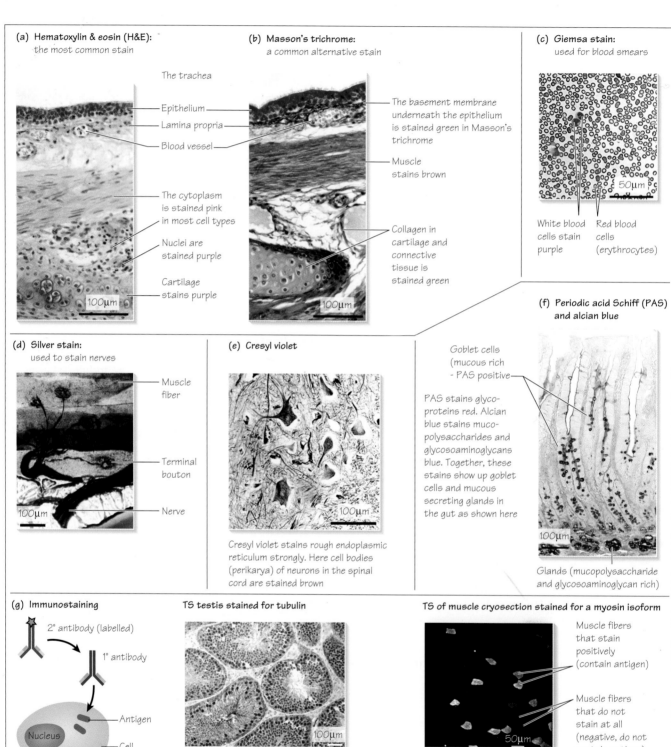

(a) Hematoxylin & eosin (H&E):
the most common stain

The trachea

- Epithelium
- Lamina propria
- Blood vessel

The cytoplasm is stained pink in most cell types

Nuclei are stained purple

Cartilage stains purple

100μm

(b) Masson's trichrome:
a common alternative stain

The basement membrane underneath the epithelium is stained green in Masson's trichrome

Muscle stains brown

Collagen in cartilage and connective tissue is stained green

100μm

(c) Giemsa stain:
used for blood smears

50μm

White blood cells stain purple

Red blood cells (erythrocytes)

(d) Silver stain:
used to stain nerves

- Muscle fiber
- Terminal bouton
- Nerve

100μm

(e) Cresyl violet

100μm

Cresyl violet stains rough endoplasmic reticulum strongly. Here cell bodies (perikarya) of neurons in the spinal cord are stained brown

(f) Periodic acid Schiff (PAS) and alcian blue

Goblet cells (mucous rich - PAS positive

PAS stains glyco-proteins red. Alcian blue stains muco-polysaccharides and glycosoaminoglycans blue. Together, these stains show up goblet cells and mucous secreting glands in the gut as shown here

100μm

Glands (mucopolysaccharide and glycosoaminoglycan rich)

(g) Immunostaining

2° antibody (labelled)

1° antibody

Antigen

Nucleus

Cell

Primary (1°) antibody recognises and binds to the antigen (specific protein). Secondary antibody (2°) recognises and binds to the primary antibody and is labelled with a dye so it can be visualised.

TS testis stained for tubulin

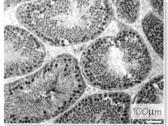

100μm

1° antibody: anti-tubulin (raised in rabbit).
2° antibody: anti-rabbit conjugated with horse-radish peroxidase (HRP). HRP is visualized using 3,3'-diaminobenzidine (DAB)+ chromagen (results in the brown staining seen here).
Blue counterstain: Mayers haemotoxylin.
Courtesy of Mohammed Abdollahi, Leeds General Infirmary

TS of muscle cryosection stained for a myosin isoform

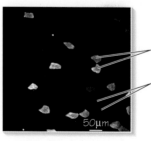

50μm

Muscle fibers that stain positively (contain antigen)

Muscle fibers that do not stain at all (negative, do not contain antigen)

1° antibody: anti-type I myosin (raised in mouse).
2° antibody: anti-mouse conjugated with a flurescent dye.
The section is visualized using epi-fluorescence microscopy

Cells are colorless and transparent, and it would be difficult to see much detail when observing them using a microscope. Therefore, stains have to be used to make the cells visible.

H&E (hematoxylin & eosin) is the most commonly used stain, but many additional stains are also used, a few of which are described here.

Hematoxylin & eosin

Hematoxylin is derived from the logwood tree (*Haematoxylum campechianum*), and can only be used as a dye in its oxidized form (hematein). It is a **basic** dye that binds to **acidic** structures in cells and stains them a purplish blue. These include:
• DNA in the nucleus, in heterochromatin and the nucleolus;
• RNA in the cytoplasm in ribosomes and rough endoplasmic reticulum;
• some extracellular materials (e.g., carbohydrates in cartilage).

Eosin is a negatively charged **acidic** dye. It binds to **basic** structures in cells and stains them red or pink. These include:
• most proteins in the cytoplasm;
• some extracellular fibers.

Cells in tissue stained with H&E (Fig. 2a) are therefore pink, with a purple nucleus.

Other types of histological stains

Connective tissue stains

Masson's trichrome method (Fig. 2b) uses three different dyes (hematoxylin, acid fuchsin, and methyl blue), resulting in three colors in the stained section.
• Nuclei are stained blue.
• Cytoplasm, red blood cells (erythrocytes), and keratin are stained bright red.
• Collagen in the basement membrane, connective tissue, and cartilage are stained green.

A related stain also used to stain connective tissue is **Van Gieson**.

Giemsa stain

This type of stain is used for bone marrow and blood smears (Fig. 2c).
• Red blood cells are stained pink (they do not have nuclei).
• White blood cells: cytoplasm is stained pale blue and the nuclei are stained dark blue/purple.

Silver staining (for neurons)

Standard histological stains do not work well on neurons, mainly because their plasma membranes are rich in lipid. Moreover, nuclei are not detected, unless the sections include part of the central nervous system, where the majority of the nuclei are located. However, **silver staining** (Fig. 2d) does work well. Silver staining stains the nerves and nerve terminals (terminal boutons)

black. An alternative method is Golgi-Cox (mercuric chloride, potassium chromate, and dichromate).

Cresyl violet

This stain is used to stain Nissl substance (rough endoplasmic reticulum; ER) in the cell bodies of neurons (Fig. 2e).

Staining carbohydrates and mucins

In the **periodic acid–Schiff (PAS) reaction,** periodic acid oxidizes carbohydrates and carbohydrate-rich molecules such as glycosaminoglycans, and the Schiff reagent stains the resultant oxidized molecules a deep reddish purple color. In the picture shown here (Fig. 2f), PAS has been combined with the dye, Alcian blue, which stains some mucins (glycosylated proteins) a deep blue color.

Goblet cells, which are rich in carbohydrates and mucin, are stained reddish purple.

Mucin-rich glands towards the bottom of the image shown here are stained a deep blue.

Stains for lipids

Lipid stains include **Oil Red O**, **Sudan black**, and **Nile blue**, and stain myelin sheaths of neurons brownish black (not shown here).

Immunocytochemistry

This technique is becoming much more widely used in histology, as it can detect specific proteins in a section. In this technique, an antibody is used that recognizes a specific antigen on the protein of interest (Fig. 2g). Usually, after incubating the section with the first antibody (primary antibody), a second antibody (secondary antibody) is added, which recognizes the primary antibody (indirect technique). The secondary antibody is commonly labeled using horseradish peroxidase, which turns brown when reacted with a chromogen substrate. This type of staining can be viewed on a normal brightfield microscope. A 'counterstain' is used to enable visualization of the overall organization of the cells in the tissue.

Alternatively, the secondary antibody is labeled with a fluorescent dye, in which case the sections have to be viewed using an epifluorescence (or confocal) microscope (see Chapter 4).

Fixing, dehydration, and wax embedding can destroy or mask antigens, which means the antibodies may not work. If this is the case, a number of different 'antigen retrieval' methods can be used, which unmask the antigens. These approaches commonly use pressure cookers or microwave ovens. Alternatively, cryosections can be used.

Staining in electron microscopy

See Chapter 4.

Sectioning and appearance of sections in the light microscope

3

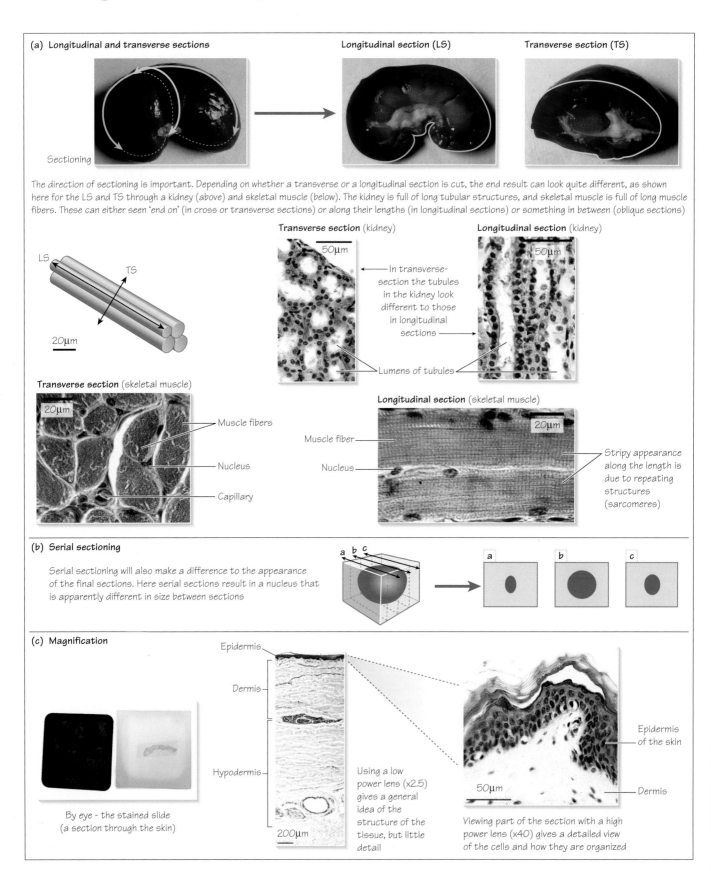

(a) Longitudinal and transverse sections

Longitudinal section (LS)

Transverse section (TS)

Sectioning

The direction of sectioning is important. Depending on whether a transverse or a longitudinal section is cut, the end result can look quite different, as shown here for the LS and TS through a kidney (above) and skeletal muscle (below). The kidney is full of long tubular structures, and skeletal muscle is full of long muscle fibers. These can either seen 'end on' (in cross or transverse sections) or along their lengths (in longitudinal sections) or something in between (oblique sections)

LS

TS

20μm

Transverse section (kidney)

50μm

In transverse-section the tubules in the kidney look different to those in longitudinal sections

Longitudinal section (kidney)

50μm

Lumens of tubules

Transverse section (skeletal muscle)

20μm

Muscle fibers

Nucleus

Capillary

Longitudinal section (skeletal muscle)

20μm

Muscle fiber

Nucleus

Stripy appearance along the length is due to repeating structures (sarcomeres)

(b) Serial sectioning

Serial sectioning will also make a difference to the appearance of the final sections. Here serial sections result in a nucleus that is apparently different in size between sections

a b c

a

b

c

(c) Magnification

Epidermis

Dermis

Hypodermis

200μm

By eye - the stained slide (a section through the skin)

Using a low power lens (x2.5) gives a general idea of the structure of the tissue, but little detail

50μm

Viewing part of the section with a high power lens (x40) gives a detailed view of the cells and how they are organized

Epidermis of the skin

Dermis

Tissues are thick, therefore the organization of cells within tissues cannot easily be visualized in the microscope. To see the detailed structure, sections have to be cut and stained and then visualized in the microscope.

The appearance of the sections depends on how the sections are cut (Fig. 3).

Longitudinal and transverse sections

A tissue cut longitudinally looks different to a tissue cut transversely (Fig. 3a).

A longitudinal section through kidney tubules shows long linear structures, with a central lumen, whereas a transverse section or cross-section through the same tubules shows round structures with a central lumen.

A longitudinal section through muscle tissue, in which the muscle fibers are long and thin, shows the repeating striated pattern along the length of the muscle fiber.

A transverse section through muscle tissue shows the polygonal shape of the fibers, with the nuclei at the edges; no striations are apparent.

Sections can also be cut obliquely, in which case the appearance is part-way between a longitudinal section and a cross-section.

Serial sections

Sections are cut in series through a tissue. The appearance of the cell and tissue will depend on where the section is cut (Fig. 3b).

Sections cut through the middle of cells look different from those cut through the edges.

Magnification

Once the section of tissue has been cut, stained, and mounted it is examined in a light microscope, using a range of different lenses, with different magnifications (Fig. 3c).

Viewing the slide by eye, does not show how the cells are organized in the tissue, but gives an overall impression of the tissue itself.

Examining the overall morphology of the section on a slide by eye usually gives a good idea of which tissue the section has been cut from.

To investigate the organization of the sectioned tissue in more detail, the slide is usually viewed in stages, starting with a low-power objective such as $\times 1.6$ or $\times 5$ or $\times 10$ to obtain an overall impression of the organization of the tissue. Finally, a high-power objective, $\times 20$, $\times 40$, $\times 63$ or $\times 100$, is used to examine the cells in detail.

Resolving power of the light microscope

The resolution of a microscope determines how close together two objects can be before they can no longer be distinguished as two separate objects.

High-power objectives tend to have a higher numerical aperture, collect more light and therefore have a higher resolving power.

The spatial resolution of a lens is determined by the resolving power of the microscope (d) in the following equation:

$$d = 0.61 \times \lambda / NA$$

where λ is the wavelength of the light in μm, and NA is the numerical aperture of the objective lens. This equation holds for microscopes where the numerical aperture of the condenser is greater than or equal to the numerical aperture of the objective.

Brightfield illumination, used to examine histology slides, commonly employs a tungsten lamp, which produces white light over a broad range of wavelengths (from 400–500 nm to 700–800 nm).

The resolving power of a $\times 40$ oil immersion lens, with an NA of 1.3, at a wavelength of 600 nm (0.6 μm), is $0.61 \times 0.6/1.3$, which is equal to 0.28 μm (280 nm).

Two objects that are closer together than this distance will not be resolved at this wavelength.

The resolving power of a low-power lens, which works in air, with an NA of 0.12 (for example) is only 3.05 μm at 600 nm.

This means that much less detail is visible at low magnification than at high magnification.

The overall magnification of the specimen depends on the magnification of the objective lens and the magnification of the eyepieces. It is important to determine this overall magnification from a calibration graticule for each objective–eyepiece lens combination that is used.

Electron microscopy gives the highest resolution, because it uses an electron beam that has a much shorter wavelength (about 0.1 nm) than visible light (see Chapter 4).

4 Light and electron microscopes

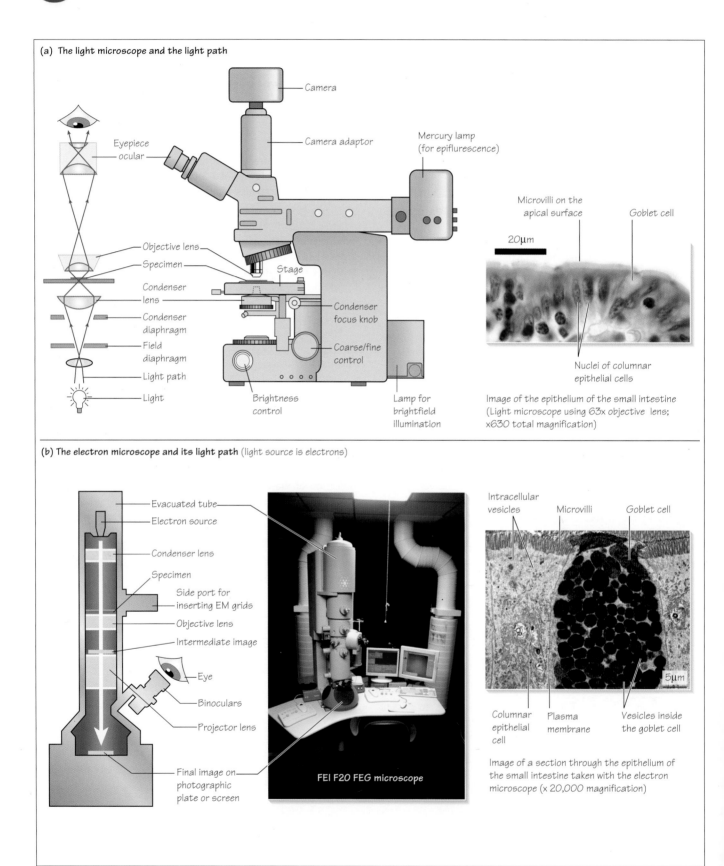

(a) The light microscope and the light path

- Camera
- Camera adaptor
- Mercury lamp (for epiflurescence)
- Eyepiece ocular
- Objective lens
- Specimen
- Stage
- Condenser lens
- Condenser diaphragm
- Field diaphragm
- Light path
- Light
- Condenser focus knob
- Coarse/fine control
- Brightness control
- Lamp for brightfield illumination

Microvilli on the apical surface
Goblet cell
20 μm
Nuclei of columnar epithelial cells

Image of the epithelium of the small intestine (Light microscope using 63x objective lens; x630 total magnification)

(b) The electron microscope and its light path (light source is electrons)

- Evacuated tube
- Electron source
- Condenser lens
- Specimen
- Side port for inserting EM grids
- Objective lens
- Intermediate image
- Eye
- Binoculars
- Projector lens
- Final image on photographic plate or screen

FEI F20 FEG microscope

Intracellular vesicles
Microvilli
Goblet cell
5 μm
Columnar epithelial cell
Plasma membrane
Vesicles inside the goblet cell

Image of a section through the epithelium of the small intestine taken with the electron microscope (x 20,000 magnification)

The light microscope

In the light microscope (Fig. 4a), illumination is provided by a tungsten lamp with a wavelength of about 400–800 nm.

Light is focused on the specimen, which is placed on the microscope stage.

The image is formed in the eyepiece by the combination of the objective lens and the eyepiece lens.

The total overall magnification depends on the magnification of both the eyepiece and the objective lens. For example, the total magnification for a ×10 eyepiece lens and a ×20 objective lens is ×200.

To obtain a clear, evenly illuminated image, it is important to set up Koehler illumination of the specimen.

In this type of illumination, all the light from the lamp is focused at the front aperture of the condenser.

Koehler illumination

Koehler illumination is achieved by:
1 focusing on the specimen;
2 closing the field diaphragm;
3 adjusting the position of the condenser to bring an image of the aperture of the field diaphragm into sharp focus;
4 opening the aperture of the diaphragm until the edges just disappear from view.

This process should be repeated each time the objective lens is changed, to ensure and bright and even illumination of the specimen.

As explained in Chapter 3, the resolution of the image depends on the lens that is used.

The very best resolution obtainable from a standard light microscope is about 0.2 μm.

Cells are about 20–40 μm in diameter, and therefore can be seen by light microscopy.

However, intracellular vesicles are usually smaller than 0.2 μm and individual vesicles cannot normally be seen by light microscopy.

The electron microscope

To investigate tissues in more detail, the electron microscope is used (Fig. 4b). The electron microscope uses an electron beam as the source of illumination, which has a much shorter wavelength than light (0.004 nm, compared to ~600 nm for light).

Electromagnetic coils are used to focus the beam, instead of lenses,

The effective numerical aperture of the electron microscope is 0.012. Therefore the theoretical resolving power (d) = $0.61 \times 0.004/0.012$ nm, or 0.2 nm.

In practice, the resolving power is less than this, due to imperfections in the electromagnetic lenses.

Usually the resolution is closer to 1 or 2 nm, and the greatest magnification is about ×50 000.

However, this means that a lot more detail can be seen by electron microscopy than by light microscopy, such as intracellular vesicles and protein filaments within cells.

The tube that the electrons move through is evacuated to reduce scatter of the electrons. This means that the samples have to be fixed before viewing in the electron microscope.

Sectioning for electron microscopy

The process of generating sections for electron microscopy is similar to that for light microscopy, but with some key differences.
1 Tissues are normally fixed with glutaraldehyde, rather than paraformaldehyde.
2 Tissues are postfixed in osmic acid.
3 As with light microscopy, the tissues are dehydrated via a series of increasing ethanol concentrations.
4 Tissues are then transferred to propylene oxide (not wax), which enables impregnation of the tissue with resin, which is allowed to harden.
5 Sections are then cut from the block using an ultramicrotome and either a glass or diamond knife. The thickness of the sections is much smaller than that for light microscopy, ranging from 60 to 100 nm thick.
6 Finally, cut sections are stained with heavy metal salts such as osmium, uranyl acetate, and lead to increase the contrast of the image, as these stains scatter the electrons.

As with light microscopy, cryosections can also be used in the electron microscope, and the sections can be immunostained, but in this case antibodies are labeled using gold, so that they are visible in the electron microscope.

5 The cell and its components

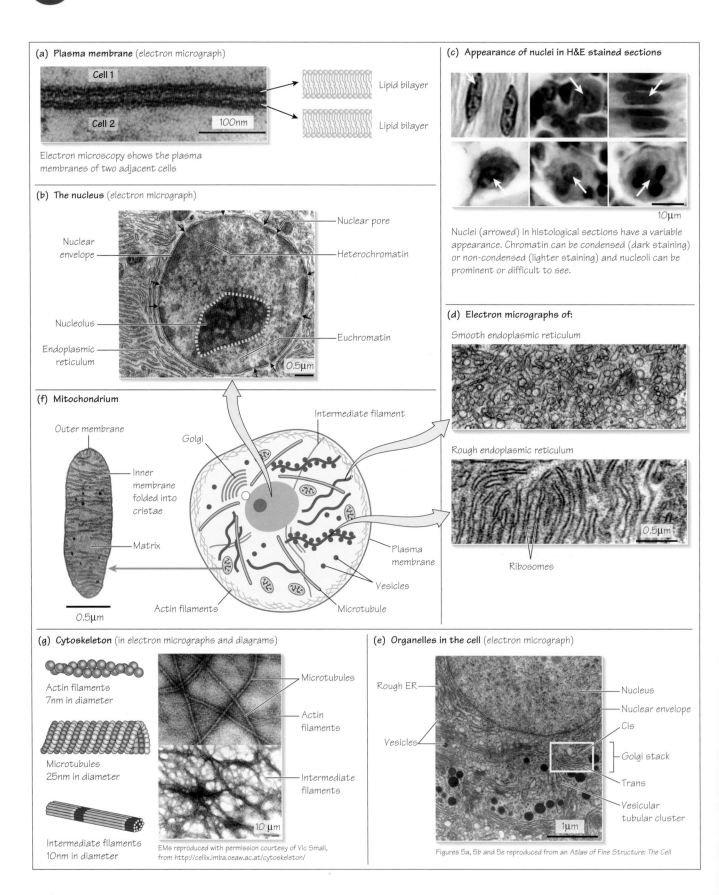

(a) Plasma membrane (electron micrograph)

Cell 1
Cell 2
100nm

Lipid bilayer
Lipid bilayer

Electron microscopy shows the plasma membranes of two adjacent cells

(b) The nucleus (electron micrograph)

Nuclear pore
Nuclear envelope
Heterochromatin
Nucleolus
Endoplasmic reticulum
Euchromatin
0.5µm

(c) Appearance of nuclei in H&E stained sections

10µm

Nuclei (arrowed) in histological sections have a variable appearance. Chromatin can be condensed (dark staining) or non-condensed (lighter staining) and nucleoli can be prominent or difficult to see.

(d) Electron micrographs of:

Smooth endoplasmic reticulum

Rough endoplasmic reticulum

0.5µm

Ribosomes

(f) Mitochondrium

Outer membrane
Inner membrane folded into cristae
Matrix
0.5µm

Golgi
Intermediate filament
Plasma membrane
Vesicles
Actin filaments
Microtubule

(g) Cytoskeleton (in electron micrographs and diagrams)

Actin filaments
7nm in diameter

Microtubules
25nm in diameter

Intermediate filaments
10nm in diameter

Microtubules
Actin filaments
Intermediate filaments

10 µm

EMs reproduced with permission courtesy of Vic Small, from http://cellix.imba.oeaw.ac.at/cytoskeleton/

(e) Organelles in the cell (electron micrograph)

Rough ER
Vesicles

Nucleus
Nuclear envelope
Cis
Golgi stack
Trans
Vesicular tubular cluster

1µm

Figures 5a, 5b and 5e reproduced from an Atlas of Fine Structure: The Cell

The plasma membrane

The plasma membrane (Fig. 5a) is the boundary between the cell and its exterior environment.

It consists of a lipid bilayer, seen by electron microscopy as two parallel electron-dense (dark) lines with a narrow gap between them.

The plasma membrane is only 8–10 nm thick, and cannot be seen by light microscopy without special dyes.

The nucleus

The nucleus (Fig. 5b), about 10 μm in diameter, is enclosed by a nuclear envelope, which forms a barrier between it and the cytoplasm. The nuclear envelope consists of both an outer and an inner nuclear membrane (lipid bilayer). Nuclear pores within the nuclear envelope control which proteins and RNA can pass between the nucleus and the cytoplasm.

Light patches of staining, known as euchromatin, contain DNA that is being actively transcribed. Darker staining patches of heterochromatin contain DNA that is not being actively transcribed. The nucleolus is where ribosomal RNA is processed and assembled into ribosome subunits.

The nucleus and the nucleoli can be seen in sections by light microscopy (Fig. 5c). The appearance of nuclei varies between cells and cell types, and depends on the activity of the cells.

Cellular organelles

Endoplasmic reticulum

The endoplasmic reticulum (ER; Fig. 5d) is a single internal membrane system that extends throughout the cytoplasm, and makes up about 10% of the total cell volume. Its membrane is continuous with the outer nuclear membrane. The ER synthesizes lipids and proteins, generating the membranes of most of the organelles in the cell, and it stores Ca^{2+}. Some proteins are internalized into its lumen and sent to the Golgi to be modified.

Rough ER (Fig. 5d) is organized into parallel layers of flattened sacs and covered with ribosomes. Its lumen is 20–30 nm wide. The cytoplasm of cells rich in rough ER stains a darker pink, or blue/purple with H&E due to the high amounts of RNA in the many ribosomes, which are acidic, and therefore stain blue/purple with hematoxylin. Rough ER synthesizes secretory proteins and lysosomal enzymes.

Smooth ER (Fig. 5d) is not covered with ribosomes. It is branched and has a wider lumen than rough ER (30–60 nm).

Golgi apparatus

The **Golgi apparatus** (Fig. 5e) is found close to the nucleus. It glycosylates proteins received from the ER and packages them for transport to the plasma membrane. It also retrieves and recycles proteins.

It consists of 3 to 7 flattened discs of membranes, called cisternae.

The receiving face of the Golgi is called the 'cis' (receiving, forming, or entry) face.

Proteins exit via the trans (maturing or exit) face.

Vesicles

Cells contain a large number of vesicles (Fig. 5e).
- **Secretory vesicles:** These travel from the Golgi to the plasma membrane.
- **Endocytic vesicles:** These travel from the plasma membrane inwards. Cells endocytose membrane proteins and extracellular material to bring them into the cell. Endocytic vesicles are called endosomes. Once inside the cell, these can fuse with vesicles called lysosomes, which break down the contents of endocytic vesicles. Cells can also endocytose fluids in larger vesicles (macropinosomes) and some cells are specialized to endocytose bacteria (phagocytosis).
- **Peroxisomes:** These degrade fatty acids by oxidation and synthesize cholesterol, and are particularly abundant in the kidney and the liver.

Vesicles are 50–200 nm in diameter and are difficult to see by light microscopy, without using special stains or immunostaining.

Mitochondria

Mitochondria (Fig. 5f; singular, mitochondrion) provide energy for the cell in the form of adenosine triphosphate (ATP). Mitochondria contain a smooth outer membrane and an inner membrane that is folded into 'christae'. Mitochondria migrate throughout the cell, can fuse, undergo fission, and can be degraded. Their appearance varies between different tissues/cells.

Cytoskeleton

There are three main types of filament in the cytoskeleton (Fig. 5g).
- **Actin filaments** (the smallest in diameter) have many cellular functions. They act as tracks for motor proteins (myosins). They facilitate cell–cell adhesion by linking the cytoskeleton to tight junctions and adherens junctions (see Chapter 7), which connect cells to each other. In addition they are key components of cellular protrusions such as microvilli.
- **Intermediate filaments** (intermediate in diameter) maintain the structural integrity of cells and facilitate cell–cell adhesion through their linkage to desmosomes and hemidesmosomes (focal adhesions; see Chapter 7). Nuclear lamins preserve the integrity of the nucleus. The type of intermediate filament is cell-type specific.
- **Microtubules** (the largest in diameter) grow out from the centrosome. These filaments act as tracks for motors (kinesins, dynein), which traffic (move) vesicles around in cells. They are also key components of cilia and flagella, and they are essential for building the mitotic (and meiotic) spindle in cell division.

6 Cell division

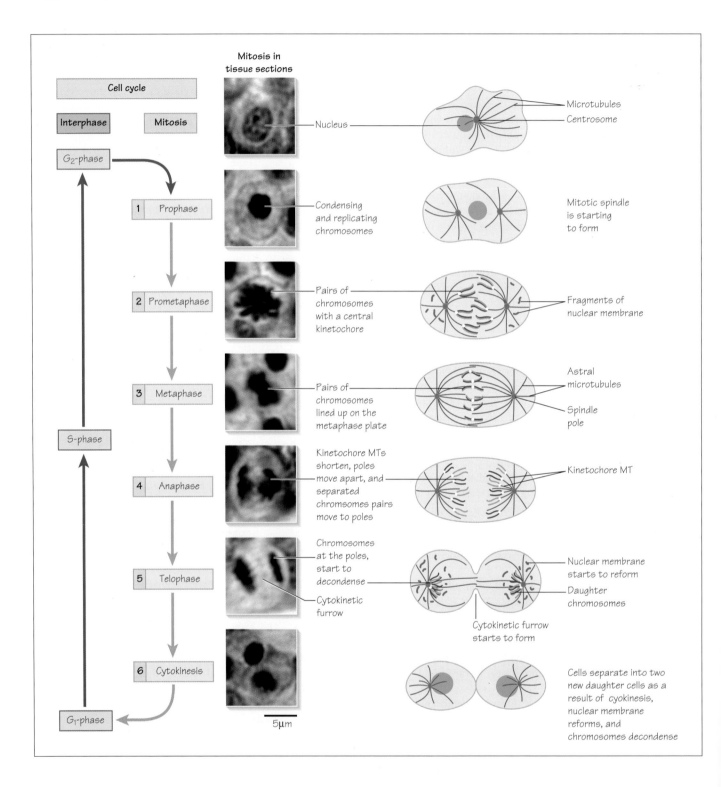

Cell cycle

Interphase — Mitosis

G_2-phase

1 Prophase

2 Prometaphase

3 Metaphase

4 Anaphase

5 Telophase

6 Cytokinesis

S-phase

G_1-phase

Mitosis in tissue sections

Nucleus

Condensing and replicating chromosomes

Pairs of chromosomes with a central kinetochore

Pairs of chromosomes lined up on the metaphase plate

Kinetochore MTs shorten, poles move apart, and separated chromsomes pairs move to poles

Chromosomes at the poles, start to decondense

Cytokinetic furrow

5μm

Microtubules

Centrosome

Mitotic spindle is starting to form

Fragments of nuclear membrane

Astral microtubules

Spindle pole

Kinetochore MT

Nuclear membrane starts to reform

Daughter chromosomes

Cytokinetic furrow starts to form

Cells separate into two new daughter cells as a result of cyokinesis, nuclear membrane reforms, and chromosomes decondense

 Histology at a Glance, 1st edition. © Michelle Peckham. Published 2011 by Blackwell Publishing Ltd.

In the cell cycle, cells spend most of their time in interphase (phase between each mitosis). Interphase is divided up into three phases:
- G_1 (growth 1): growth phase 1;
- S (synthesis): DNA replication;
- G_2 (growth 2): growth phase 2.

Following G_2, the cells can then enter mitosis.

Some cells enter G_0 after mitosis: a resting/quiescent/senescent stage, in which cells have stopped dividing.

Many cells in the body are terminally differentiated, and do not divide, an example being skeletal muscle. Therefore, you will not commonly find examples of dividing cells in tissue sections, but they can be seen occasionally, depending on the tissue.

Mitosis

Each cell contains two pairs of chromosomes, one of which is paternally, and one maternally derived.

Cell division occurs about once every 24–48 hours in cells that have not yet terminally differentiated. Cell division only takes about 30–60 minutes. Dividing cells can sometimes be observed in tissue sections and are often called 'mitotic figures'. The different phases of cell division can be identified in tissue sections (Fig. 6).

Prophase

In prophase (Fig. 6, stage 1), the centrosome duplicates and the two resultant centrosomes move apart to form the poles of the mitotic spindle. The replicated chromosomes condense, and associate (sister chromatids). They are held together along their length. Pairs of paternal and maternal chromosomes remain separate.

Prometaphase

In prometaphase (Fig. 6, stage 2), the nuclear membrane breaks down, and the spindle is formed. There are three main types of microtubules.
- Astral microtubules: These grow out from the poles to towards the plasma membrane anchoring the spindle in the center of the cell.
- Kinetochore microtubules: These grow out from the poles and attach to the kinetochores of the chromosomes.
- Spindle microtubules: These can attach to the arms of chromosomes.

Chromosome movement is highly dynamic during this stage.

Metaphase

In metaphase (Fig. 6, stage 3), all the chromosomes become aligned on the metaphase plate. Each chromosome pair is attached to kinetochore microtubules from each of the two poles.

Anaphase

In anaphase (Fig. 6, stage 4), when each pair of chromosomes is aligned on the metaphase plate (spindle checkpoint), the kinetochore microtubules rapidly shorten, and together with molecular motors (kinesin and dynein) the pairs of chromosomes are separated. Each half of the pair (daughter chromosome) is moved apart to the poles very rapidly. In the second stage of anaphase, the poles move outwards towards the plasma membrane. This phase is very rapid (takes a few minutes).

Telophase

In telophase (Fig. 6, stage 5), the pairs of chromosomes have fully separated. The daughter chromosomes are found at the poles of the spindle. The nuclear envelope starts to reform, and the cytokinetic furrow starts to form.

Cytokinesis

In cytokinesis (Fig. 6, stage 6), the cytokinetic furrow pinches off the two cells from each other. The nuclear envelope has reformed, and the DNA in the chromosomes has condensed.

Mitosis is exquisitely controlled. In particular, the metaphase checkpoint is used to make sure all the pairs of chromosomes are lined up at the metaphase plate, before they are separated. Problems in mitosis can result in cells that contain an abnormal number of chromosomes, either losing or gaining chromosomes (aneuploidy). This can result in pre-cancerous cells (cancer 'stem' cells).

Meiosis

Meiosis is similar to mitosis but with several important differences (not shown here).
- There are two sets of meiotic divisions, resulting in 4 haploid cells, rather than one division resulting in 2 diploid cells.
- Prophase I: In prophase of the first meiotic division, pairs of homologous chromosomes (maternal and paternal) adhere together to form bivalents (In mitosis, each pair of homologous chromosomes remains separate.)
- During this stage, crossovers between maternal and paternal chromosomes can occur. About 2–3 crossovers per chromosome occur in humans. This process is important for generating genetic diversity.
- Metaphase I: The bivalents line up on the metaphase plate.
- Anaphase I: Sister chromatids separate and chromosomes are segregated into daughter cells, such that one cell will inherit the paternal homolog and the other the maternal homolog, for each chromosome.
- Meiosis II: A second meiotic division separates the sister chromatids, resulting in haploid cells.

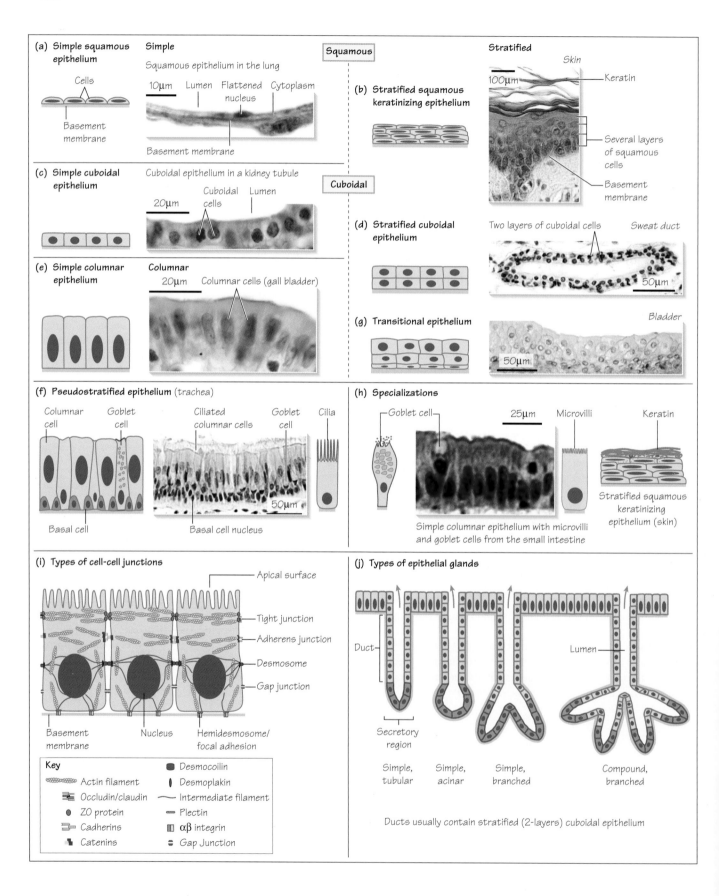

(a) **Simple squamous epithelium**

Cells

Basement membrane

Simple

Squamous epithelium in the lung

10μm | Lumen | Flattened nucleus | Cytoplasm

Basement membrane

(c) **Simple cuboidal epithelium**

Cuboidal epithelium in a kidney tubule

20μm | Cuboidal cells | Lumen

(e) **Simple columnar epithelium**

Columnar

20μm | Columnar cells (gall bladder)

Squamous

Cuboidal

(b) **Stratified squamous keratinizing epithelium**

Stratified

Skin

100μm — Keratin

Several layers of squamous cells

Basement membrane

(d) **Stratified cuboidal epithelium**

Two layers of cuboidal cells | Sweat duct

50μm

(g) **Transitional epithelium**

Bladder

50μm

(f) **Pseudostratified epithelium** (trachea)

Columnar cell | Goblet cell

Ciliated columnar cells | Goblet cell | Cilia

Basal cell

Basal cell nucleus

50μm

(h) **Specializations**

Goblet cell | 25μm | Microvilli | Keratin

Simple columnar epithelium with microvilli and goblet cells from the small intestine

Stratified squamous keratinizing epithelium (skin)

(i) **Types of cell-cell junctions**

Apical surface

Tight junction

Adherens junction

Desmosome

Gap junction

Basement membrane | Nucleus | Hemidesmosome/ focal adhesion

Key

- Actin filament
- Occludin/claudin
- ZO protein
- Cadherins
- Catenins
- Desmocoilin
- Desmoplakin
- Intermediate filament
- Plectin
- αβ integrin
- Gap Junction

(j) **Types of epithelial glands**

Duct

Lumen

Secretory region

Simple, tubular | Simple, acinar | Simple, branched | Compound, branched

Ducts usually contain stratified (2-layers) cuboidal epithelium

Functions of epithelium

The epithelium covers or lines all of the internal and external body surfaces (i.e., skin, nasal cavity, gut, etc).

The epithelium acts as a barrier, controlling:
• diffusion across the epithelium;
• absorption by epithelial cells;
• secretion of substances onto the outside of the epithelium.

The epithelium also provides physical protection.

The epithelium consists of a continuous sheet of one or more layers of cells that are tightly connected to each other, and to the underlying layer of connective tissue (the basement membrane). The epithelium is **avascular**. Cells rely on diffusion across the basement membrane for their nourishment.

Classification of epithelium

Epithelium is classified as either:
• **simple** (one layer of cells); or
• **stratified** (two or more layers of cells);
and on the basis of cell shape as either:
• **squamous**: contains flat cells (width is much greater than the height). This facilitates transport and rapid diffusion across the epithelium.
• **cuboidal**: square/cuboidal cell shape. These cells usually active in excretion, secretion or absorption, and the Golgi and organelles lie between the nucleus and the apical surface.
• **columnar**: height is greater than width. These cells are highly active in secretion.

A **simple squamous epithelium** (Fig. 7a) lines the lungs, and all blood vessels (where it is called the **endothelium**), and forms the **mesothelial** lining of all the body cavities.

A **stratified squamous epithelium** (Fig. 7b) protects against abrasion. Examples include the epithelium of skin and the oesophagus.

A **simple cuboidal epithelium** (Fig. 7c) lines secretory regions of some glands, and tubules in the kidney.

A **stratified cuboidal epithelium** (Fig. 7d) lines the excretory regions of glands, e.g., the sweat glands of skin.

A **simple columnar epithelium** (Fig. 7e) lines the stomach (and the gall bladder).

Pseudostratified epithelium

This is a simple epithelium that looks stratified (Fig. 7f) because the nuclei of the cells that make up this type of epithelium are found at different levels, giving it a stratified appearance. It contains columnar cells that span from the basement membrane to the lumen, and smaller basal cells (stem cells that renew the epithelium) with basally located nuclei.

Transitional epithelium

This is a stratified epithelium (Fig. 7g) in which the cells change their appearance, appearing cuboidal in relaxed epithelium and squamous when the epithelium is stretched.

Specializations of the epithelium

• **Microvilli:** small thin protrusions on the apical surface of cells, which contain bundles of actin filaments, and increase the surface area of the cell for absorption (Fig. 7h).
• **Cilia:** long fine projections on the apical surface that contain a core of microtubules. Motile cilia beat rhythmically, moving mucus on the apical surface of cells (Fig. 7f).
• **Goblet cells:** Specialized epithelial cells that secrete mucus (glygoproteins and proteoglycans) onto the apical surface of the epithelium. These are single 'glandular' cells (Fig. 7h).
• **Keratin:** found on the outer surfaces of epithelia that experience abrasion and water loss. Keratin is a type of intermediate filament, which is made and secreted by epithelial cells in a highly crosslinked form onto the outermost surface (Fig. 7h).

Connections within the epithelium

Four main types of junction (Fig. 7i) connect epithelial cells to each other.
• **Tight junctions** are close to the apical surface.
• **Adherens junctions** are just below the apical surface. Both tight and adherens junctions involve actin filaments.
• **Desmosomes** involve intermediate filaments.
• **Gap junctions** are communicating junctions (not structural) for communication.

These cell–cell junctions are important for maintaining the integrity of the epithelium.

Hemidesmosomes (focal adhesions) are junctions/connections that connect the basal layer of the epithelium to the underlying basement membrane.

Epithelial glands

Epithelial cells can become specialized to form glands (Fig. 7j). These are either:
• **exocrine** glands (secretions released via ducts); or
• **endocrine** glands (ductless; secretions released directly into the bloodstream).

Exocrine glands are classified as:
• simple (unbranched duct); or
• compound (branched ducts).

Secretory regions of glands can either be:
• tubular (alveolar, e.g., sweat glands) or
• acinar (shaped like a grape, e.g., salivary glands).

Secretions are released via:
• exocytosis (**merocrine** secretion, i.e. sweat glands);
• rupture of the entire cell, and release of its products (**holocrine**, i.e. sebaceous glands);
• a mixture of the above (**apocrine**, a third rare type of secretion).

Secretions can either be:
• **serous** (watery);
• **mucous** (viscid, contains glycoproteins); or
• a mixture of the two.

8 Skeletal muscle

(a) Diagram of a cross section through a muscle fibre: three layers of connective tissue

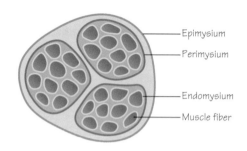

- Epimysium
- Perimysium
- Endomysium
- Muscle fiber

(c) Skeletal muscle (LS)

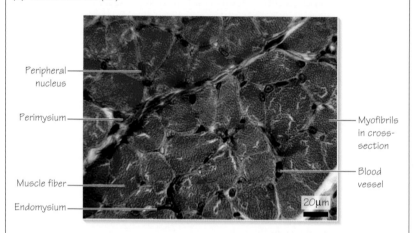

20μm

Cross-wise striations — Endomysium

Myofibrils run longitudinally along the muscle fiber

Capillary

Peripheral nucleus

The cross striations are due to the regular repeating units along the muscle fiber called 'muscle sarcomeres'

(b) Skeletal muscle fibers are formed by fusion of many myoblasts

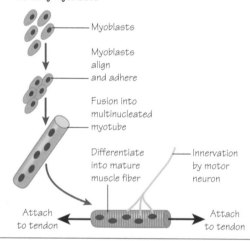

- Myoblasts
- Myoblasts align and adhere
- Fusion into multinucleated myotube
- Differentiate into mature muscle fiber
- Innervation by motor neuron

Attach to tendon ← → Attach to tendon

(d) Skeletal Muscle (TS)

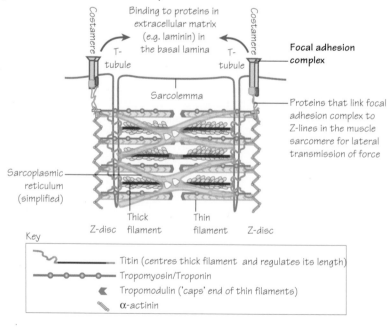

- Peripheral nucleus
- Perimysium
- Muscle fiber
- Endomysium
- Myofibrils in cross-section
- Blood vessel

20μm

(e) Electron micrograph of a sarcomere

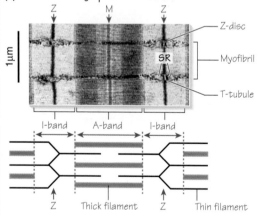

Z   M   Z

1μm

- Z-disc
- Myofibril
- SR
- T-tubule

I-band   A-band   I-band

Z   Thick filament   Z   Thin filament

The muscle sarcomere

In cardiac and skeletal muscle cells, thick (myosin-containing) filaments and thin (actin-containing) filaments are organized into regular repeating units called the muscle sarcomere. A single sarcomere extends from one Z-disc to the next. The stripes in H&E stained longitudinal sections shown above (1c) show the end-to-end arrangement of many muscle sarcomeres along the fiber. Reproduced from Skeletal Muscle, Henning Schmalbruch (1986), Springer Verlag. With kind permission of Springer Science+Business Media

(f) A sarcomere and some of its components

Costamere   Costamere

Binding to proteins in extracellular matrix (e.g. laminin) in the basal lamina

T-tubule   T-tubule

Focal adhesion complex

Sarcolemma

Proteins that link focal adhesion complex to Z-lines in the muscle sarcomere for lateral transmission of force

Sarcoplasmic reticulum (simplified)

Thick filament   Thin filament

Z-disc   Z-disc

Key

- Titin (centres thick filament and regulates its length)
- Tropomyosin/Troponin
- Tropomodulin ('caps' end of thin filaments)
- α-actinin

Skeletal muscles move joints, support the skeleton, and assist in breathing. They are connected to the skeleton via tendons, and they are all under voluntary control.

Skeletal muscle fibers are arranged into bundles (fascicles) and muscle contains three connective tissue layers (Fig. 8a):
- **epimysium:** an outer layer around the muscle;
- **perimysium:** surrounds each fiber bundle (fascicle);
- **endomysium:** surrounds each fiber.

Each muscle fiber is also surrounded by its own basal lamina.

Muscle structure and contraction

Skeletal muscle fibers are the largest cells in the body, with a single cell stretching from one end of the muscle to the other. Given the lengths of skeletal muscles, this means a single fiber (up to about 100 μm in diameter) can be several centimeters long.

Skeletal muscle fibers can be this large, because they contain thousands of nuclei, which are required to maintain a cell of this size. Thus muscle fibers are single, **multinucleated** cells. The **nuclei** are found at the **cell periphery**, and there is approximately one nucleus every 35 μm along the fiber length.

Multinucleated skeletal muscle fibers are formed by the fusion of many mononucleated cells (myoblasts) together during development, and growth (Fig. 8b).

In longitudinal sections, muscle fibers have a stripy appearance (Fig. 8c). These stripes result from the arrangement of repeating units called **sarcomeres** in series along the fiber. In skeletal muscle, sarcomeres are about 2.5 μm long. A fiber, 30 cm long, contains 120 thousand sarcomeres arranged end to end.

Sarcomeres are arranged longitudinally in structures called myofibrils (Fig. 8c), which are about 1 μm thick. Myofibrils pack together laterally in the muscle fiber, with their Z-lines aligned and connected to each other. The myofibrils can also be seen in cross-section (Fig. 8d) as punctate structures.

At the plasma membrane, the Z-lines are connected to structures called **costameres** by a number of different proteins. Transmembrane proteins (e.g., integrins) in the costameres bind to extracellular proteins in the basal lamina (e.g., laminin). This series of lateral connections enables force to be transmitted laterally through to the extracellular matrix (Fig. 8f).

The structure of the sarcomere can be seen more clearly by electron microscopy (Fig. 8e). Each sarcomere is bordered by a structure called the Z-disc. Myosin and actin are organized into thick and thin filaments, respectively, in the muscle sarcomeres (Fig. 8f).

During contraction, each sarcomere shortens by about 0.1 to 0.2 μm, and this is summed along the length of the fiber, such that the ends of the muscle shorten by a few centimeters.

Longitudinally, muscle fibers are connected via tendons at the ends of the muscles to the skeleton, to generate movement of joints.

Diseases such as congenital myopathies can affect the normal organization of actin into thin filaments. This results in a decrease in muscle mass, as well as disorganized muscle sarcomeres. This disease can result in severe muscle weakness, such that babies born with a severe form of this condition are unable to breathe unaided.

Activation of muscle contraction

Muscle fibers are innervated by nerves, which form a connection with the muscle fiber called the neuromuscular junction (NMJ; see Chapter 11).

Acetylcholine released by the NMJ binds to receptors in the postsynaptic membrane of the skeletal muscle fibers, resulting in their depolarization. Skeletal muscle (and cardiac muscle) contains **T-tubules**, which are invaginations of the plasma membrane or sarcolemma). The t-tubules are in direct contact with the internal membrane system called the **sarcoplasmic reticulum** (SR) at structures known as triads. Proteins, such as the ryanodine receptor, span between the T-tubules and the SR to facilitate this connection. The SR contains the main internal store of Ca^{2+}. When skeletal or cardiac muscle is stimulated to contract, T-tubules are depolarized, and Ca^{2+} is released from the SR into the cytoplasm. Ca^{2+} release is facilitated by the ryanodine receptor.

Once released into the cytoplasm, Ca^{2+} binds to a subunit of troponin (troponin-C), which is present on the thin, actin-containing filaments. This results in the movement of tropomyosin around the thin filament, which exposes sites on actin to which myosin cross-bridges bind. The cross-bridges then bind to actin and generate force or movement, using ATP hydrolysis to power their motion. The muscle relaxes, when Ca^{2+} levels fall back to low levels, which is achieved by pumping Ca^{2+} back into the SR.

Mutations in the ryanodine receptor cause the disease, malignant hyperthermia. In this disease, patients suffer symptoms that include muscle contractures, increased heart rate, and rapid increase in body temperature, when under general anesthesia using volatile anesthetics. This can result in the death of a patient while under anesthesia.

Muscle damage and repair

Muscle fibers are terminally differentiated and do not undergo mitosis. However, 'satellite' cells, which are skeletal muscle 'stem cells', can repair damaged muscle fibers. These cells lie under the basal lamina of the muscle fibers. When the muscle is damaged, they are stimulated to divide to generate new myoblasts, which fuse and repair the damaged muscle fiber. Skeletal muscle is most susceptible to damage as a result of eccentric exercise (actively contracting a muscle, during lengthening).

9 | Cardiac and smooth muscle

(a) Cardiac muscle (LS, iron hematoxylin stain)

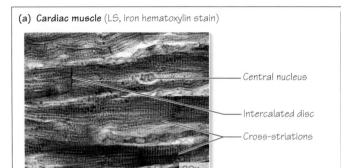

— Central nucleus

— Intercalated disc

— Cross-striations

20μm

(b) Cardiac muscle (TS, iron hematoxylin stain)

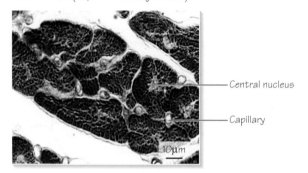

— Central nucleus

— Capillary

10μm

(c) EM of cardiac muscle showing intercalated disc

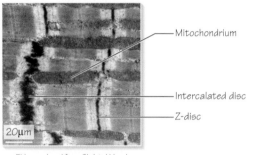

— Mitochondrium

— Intercalated disc

— Z-disc

20μm

EM reproduced from *Skeletal Muscle*,
Henning Schmalbruch, (1986) Springer Verlag, with
kind permission of Springer Science+Business Media

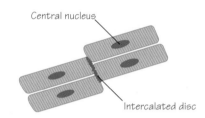

Central nucleus

Intercalated disc

Cardiac muscle cells (about 100 μm long) have a single centrally located nucleus. They are tightly connected to each other by intercalated discs and can make branching connections with more than one cell

(d) Smooth muscle (LS, modified hematoxylin stain)

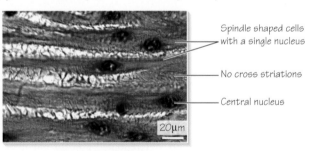

— Spindle shaped cells with a single nucleus

— No cross striations

— Central nucleus

20μm

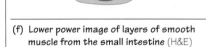

(e) Smooth muscle (TS)

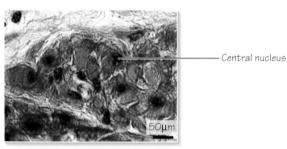

— Central nucleus

50μm

Smooth muscle cells are spindle shaped, and have a single centrally localized nucleus. They are attached to each other by desmosomes, and communicate by gap junctions. Here the cells have shrunk slightly due to processing, and the connections between the cells can be seen

(f) Lower power image of layers of smooth muscle from the small intestine (H&E)

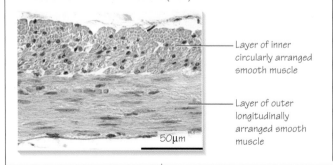

— Layer of inner circularly arranged smooth muscle

— Layer of outer longitudinally arranged smooth muscle

50μm

(g) Layers of circumferentially arranged smooth muscle cells around the lumen of a blood vessel

50μm

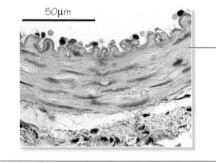

— Smooth muscle layer around a blood vessel

Cardiac muscle

This type of muscle is found in the myocardium of the heart, and is 'involuntary'. It is innervated by the regular pacemaker activity of the sino-atrial node.

Cardiac muscle is made up of a functional syncytium of cells that only have **one nucleus** (occasionally two), which is **centrally localized** (Fig. 9a,b).

These cells are called **cardiomyocytes**.

Structure and excitation of cardiomyocytes

Similar to skeletal muscle fibers, cardiomyocytes have a striated (stripy) appearance, which arises from the regular arrangement of actin-containing thin filaments and myosin-containing thick filaments in muscle sarcomeres (Fig. 9a). Resting sarcomere length in cardiac muscle (about 2.2 μm) is slightly shorter than that in skeletal muscle.

Cardiomyocytes are much smaller (about 80–100 μm long and about 15 μm in diameter) than skeletal muscle fibers.

Intercalated discs connect the cardiomyocytes to each other (Fig. 9a,c). These structures contain adherens junctions and desmosomes, which tightly connect adjacent cells, and gap junctions.

The gap junctions electrically couple the cardiomyocytes, enabling the rapid spread of contraction around the heart.

This tight structural and electrical connectivity results in the functional syncytium.

Although not directly stimulated by a nerve, cardiac cells are stimulated to contract by the influx of Ca^{2+} ions as a result of T-tubule depolarization, release of Ca^{2+} from the sarcoplasmic reticulum (SR) and the uptake of Ca^{2+} from the extracellular space.

Growth and repair

Cardiac muscle cells can hypertrophy (grow larger) or hypotrophy (grow smaller) as a result of changing demands on the heart, but the cells are terminally differentiated and cannot divide.

The heart does not appear to contain large numbers of 'stem' cells similar to the satellite cells of skeletal muscle, and therefore only has a limited ability to regenerate when damaged.

Smooth muscle

Structure and excitation of smooth muscle cells

Smooth muscle contains spindle-shaped cells, with a central nucleus, that are connected together in a functional syncytium (Fig. 9d–g). Desmosomes connect the cells together structurally, and gap junctions connect the cells electrically and chemically.

These cells **do not** have a striated appearance because they **do not** contain muscle sarcomeres. Instead, arrays of actin filaments, connected to dense bodies, surround myosin filaments in a less well-organized fashion.

The dense bodies are connected to the plasma membrane by intermediate filaments, which transmit the force generated by the interaction of actin and myosin and enable the whole cell to contract.

The SR is much reduced in this muscle.

Contraction is activated by Ca^{2+}, which mainly enters through ion channels from the extracellular space.

The Ca^{2+} influx activates myosin light chain kinase, which phosphorylates the myosin molecules in the thick filaments and activates them so that they can then interact with actin. (Thin filaments in smooth muscle do not contain troponin.) The muscle relaxes when myosin is dephosphorylated. This type of muscle generates long, slow, contractions.

Myoepithelial cells are single smooth muscle cells that surround ducts or blood vessels, and lie within the basement membrane. When these cells contract, they squeeze the ducts, helping to extrude the contents.

Growth and repair

Of all the muscle types, smooth muscle cells have the greatest capacity for regeneration. They can divide and increase in number. Numerous cells called pericytes, which lie along the small blood vessels, can divide and generate new smooth muscle cells. Smooth muscle cells can also hypertrophy.

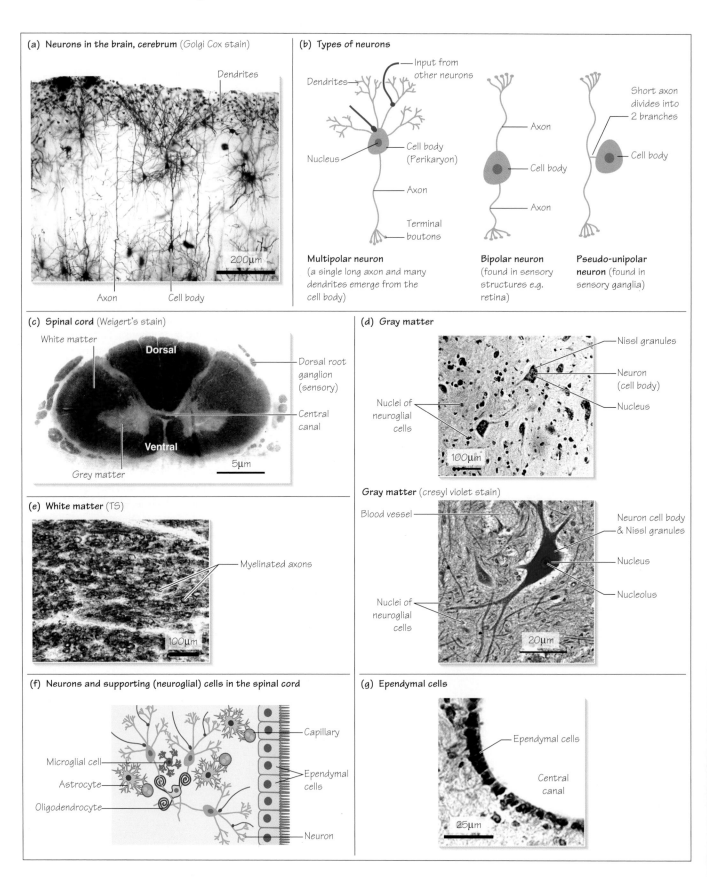

(a) Neurons in the brain, cerebrum (Golgi Cox stain)

Dendrites

Axon   Cell body

200µm

(b) Types of neurons

Input from other neurons

Dendrites

Nucleus

Cell body (Perikaryon)

Axon

Terminal boutons

Multipolar neuron (a single long axon and many dendrites emerge from the cell body)

Axon

Cell body

Axon

Bipolar neuron (found in sensory structures e.g. retina)

Short axon divides into 2 branches

Cell body

Pseudo-unipolar neuron (found in sensory ganglia)

(c) Spinal cord (Weigert's stain)

White matter

Dorsal

Ventral

Grey matter

Dorsal root ganglion (sensory)

Central canal

5µm

(d) Gray matter

Nuclei of neuroglial cells

Nissl granules

Neuron (cell body)

Nucleus

100µm

Gray matter (cresyl violet stain)

Blood vessel

Nuclei of neuroglial cells

Neuron cell body & Nissl granules

Nucleus

Nucleolus

20µm

(e) White matter (TS)

Myelinated axons

100µm

(f) Neurons and supporting (neuroglial) cells in the spinal cord

Microglial cell

Astrocyte

Oligodendrocyte

Capillary

Ependymal cells

Neuron

(g) Ependymal cells

Ependymal cells

Central canal

25µm

The **central nervous system** (CNS) consists of the brain and spinal cord. It contains gray and white matter (see below) made up of neurons and supporting cells.

The CNS is derived from surface ectoderm in the embryo, which folds up into a hollow cylinder (the neural tube).

The **somatic nervous system** controls voluntary functions and the **autonomic nervous system** involuntary functions.

Neurons

Many neurons (nerve cells) are very long and not easy to see in a single section. However, smaller neurons in the cerebrum can be seen (Fig. 10a), using heavy metal staining and thick sections. They consist of a cell body (perikaryon, or soma), a single axon and several dendrites. They range in diameter from 0.2 to 20 µm. They conduct electrical impulses.

The cell bodies of most neurons are located in the CNS. A few lie just outside the spinal cord in the ganglia, which are part of the peripheral nervous system (PNS).

The cell body contains the nucleus and is rich in Golgi, mitochondria, and rough endoplasmic reticulum (ER), also known as Nissl bodies. Proteins and mRNA are trafficked to and from the cell body along the axon along microtubules, using microtubule motors. Kinesins generally traffic substances away from the cell body and dyneins traffic substances back to the cell body.

There are **three main types of neuron** (Fig. 10b).
• **Multipolar neuron:** most common. Multiple short extensions of the cell body (dendrites), receive input from other neurons, and a single longer extension (axon), which transmits impulses to other neurons, or targets such as muscle.
• **Bipolar neuron:** a single axon and a single dendrite. Specialized neurons involved in sight, smell, and balance.
• **Pseudounipolar neuron:** a single axon and dendrite, which arise from a common stem. These are primary sensory neurons.

Synapses

Neurons make **synapses** (connections) with other neurons, or with their target organs (e.g., a muscle fiber) (see Chapter 11).

Synapses can form:
• between two axons (axoaxonic);
• between an axon and a dendrite (axodendritic); or
• between an axon and a cell body (axosomatic).

Electrical synapses (rare) are formed between two neurons, and the nerve impulse is transmitted directly via conduction of ions through gap junctions.

Chemical synapses (more common; see Chapter 10) connect neurons with their target organs, or neurons to other neurons.

Groups of neurons can be organized into:
• **layers** (strata), e.g., in the cerebral cortex;
• **bundles** (tracts or fasciculi), e.g., optic tract;
• **ganglia**, e.g., in the peripheral nervous system (PNS).

Axons of motor neurons exit the spinal cord in the nerves, and form synapses with their target organs such as skeletal muscle.

White and gray matter

A section through the spinal cord shows the central 'gray' matter surrounded by 'white' matter (Fig. 10c).
• **Gray matter** (Fig. 10d) contains all the cell bodies (**perikarya** or **soma**) of neurons, their unmyelinated dendrites, and all the cells that support the neurons (**neuroglia**).
• **White matter** (Fig. 10e) contains myelinated neurons, and a small number of cell bodies (from supporting cells only).

Supporting cells in the central nervous system (neuroglia)

Supporting cells (Fig. 10f) are the most common type of cell in the CNS and, unlike neurons, they are able to undergo mitosis, and proliferate.
• **Astrocytes** are the most common type of supporting cell, and are mostly found in white matter. They make connections called 'end-feet' with capillaries, and they facilitate metabolic exchange between neurons and blood. They are star-shaped in appearance, when stains are used that show up the cell body and all its processes. They are derived from the neuroectoderm.
• **Oligodendrocytes** generate the myelin sheath for up to 50 axons. The myelin sheath (similar to that formed by Schwann cells in the PNS) insulates the nerve and increases the rate at which the axon conducts its action potential. In the disease, multiple sclerosis, the myelin sheath is damaged, and axons become demyelinated. Oligodendrocytes are derived from the neuroectoderm.
• **Microglia** (less common) play a role in immune defense, and can become phagocytic. These cells are derived from the mesoderm.

These three types of cells are difficult to distinguish in routine histological sections, but they can be distinguished by immunocytochemistry, using antibodies that recognize proteins specific to each cell type.
• **Ependymal cells** (Fig. 10g) make up the ependyma, which lines the ventricles of the brain and the central canal of the spinal cord. They contain microvilli and one or more cilia on their apical (lumenal) surface, and are made up of a tightly connected simple cuboidal epithelium.

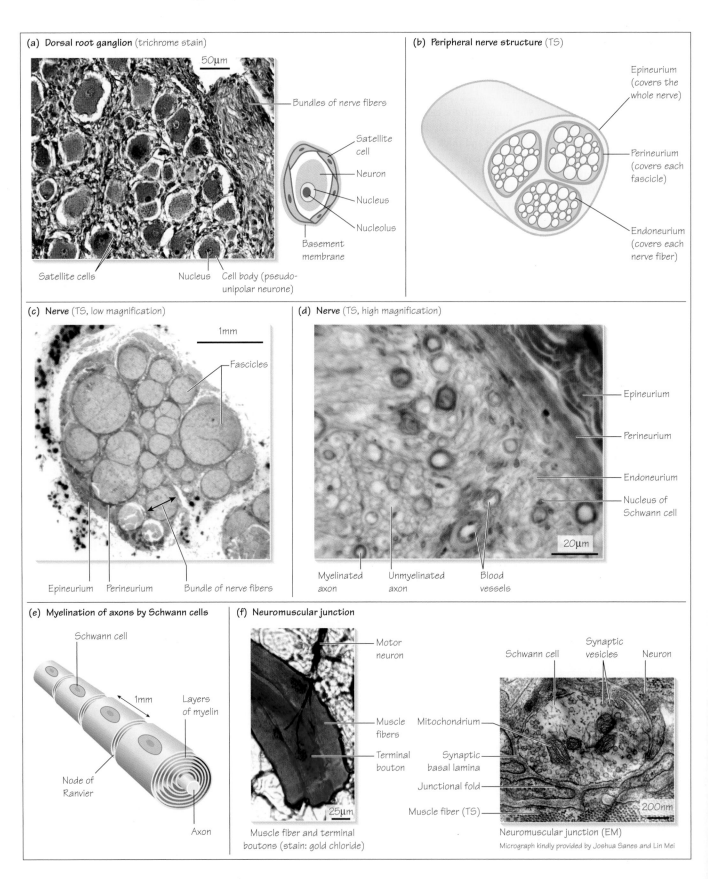

(a) Dorsal root ganglion (trichrome stain)

50μm

Bundles of nerve fibers

Satellite cell

Neuron

Nucleus

Nucleolus

Basement membrane

Satellite cells

Nucleus

Cell body (pseudo-unipolar neurone)

(b) Peripheral nerve structure (TS)

Epineurium (covers the whole nerve)

Perineurium (covers each fascicle)

Endoneurium (covers each nerve fiber)

(c) Nerve (TS, low magnification)

1mm

Fascicles

Epineurium   Perineurium   Bundle of nerve fibers

(d) Nerve (TS, high magnification)

Epineurium

Perineurium

Endoneurium

Nucleus of Schwann cell

20μm

Myelinated axon   Unmyelinated axon   Blood vessels

(e) Myelination of axons by Schwann cells

Schwann cell

1mm

Layers of myelin

Node of Ranvier

Axon

(f) Neuromuscular junction

Motor neuron

Muscle fibers

Terminal bouton

25μm

Muscle fiber and terminal boutons (stain: gold chloride)

Schwann cell

Synaptic vesicles

Neuron

Mitochondrium

Synaptic basal lamina

Junctional fold

Muscle fiber (TS)

200nm

Neuromuscular junction (EM)

Micrograph kindly provided by Joshua Sanes and Lin Mei

The **peripheral nervous system** (PNS) consists of all the nervous tissue outside the CNS, including cranial nerves, spinal nerves, and ganglia.

Nerve ganglia

These are nodular masses of neuronal cell bodies, together with their supporting neuroglia found just outside the CNS (e.g., dorsal root ganglia (Fig. 11a), which lie just outside the spinal cord, and cranial ganglia, in the head). They contain:

• **sensory neurons** in the **dorsal root** and **cranial ganglia** in the PNS;
• **sympathetic** and **parasympathetic motor neurons** in **autonomic ganglia** (PNS);
• **satellite cells**: epithelial Schwann-like cells that surround the neuron, and rest on a basement membrane are found in ganglia as shown here (Fig. 11a).

The neurons in the ganglia are derived from neural crest cells, which originate from a region just above the neural tube in the embryo.

The **dorsal root ganglia** contain the cell bodies of sensory neurons (sensory ganglia) and the cell bodies of afferent neurons from the autonomic nervous system. These neurons are pseudo-unipolar, and the fascicles of the nerves are myelinated.

The **sympathetic (autonomic) ganglia** contain multipolar neurons, most of which are not myelinated. They receive axons from presynaptic cells in the CNS.

Peripheral nerve structure

Neurons are bundled into **fascicles** inside nerves. There are three types of connective tissue coverings (Fig. 11b).

• **Endoneurium**: covers each neuron (nerve fiber) and its associated Schwann cells. It consists of bundles of collagen fibrils that run parallel to and around the nerve fibers. Endoneurium is secreted by a few fibroblasts and the Schwann cells.
• **Perineurium**: covers a bundles of fibers in a fascicle. It contains concentric layers of fibroblasts, which are tightly connected to each other by tight junctions, and which are surrounded by a basal lamina. This generates a protective 'blood–nerve' barrier, which only allows selected substances to pass across the barrier, and is analogous to the blood–brain barrier in the brain. This barrier is important in controlling diffusion of substances from the blood into the brain. It allows free transport of glucose and other selected molecules, but most substances cannot cross this barrier.
• **Epineurium**: covers the whole nerve (Fig. 11c,d), and is an example of dense connective tissue.

Supporting cells

Schwann cells are the main type of supporting cell in the PNS (Fig. 11e).

Schwann cells wrap their plasma membrane concentrically around the axon, forming a segment of myelin sheath about 1 mm long. One Schwann cell generates the myelin sheath around the axon between each node of Ranvier.

These tightly wrapped myelin layers are difficult to see in H&E sections due to their high lipid content, which is extracted by the tissue processing procedure. However, they can be seen if a stain such as osmium is combined with H&E (Fig. 11c,d).

Small gaps between each segment of sheath (nodes of Ranvier) allow saltatory conduction (the propagation of nerve impulses from one node to the next; Fig. 11e).

In **myelinated** axons, an individual Schwann cell envelops a single axon multiple times (Fig. 11d,e).

In so-called **unmyelinated** axons, in fact the axons are myelinated, but a single Schwann cell envelopes several axons, and does not form tightly wrapped layers around the axon. Instead the axons sit in grooves in the surfaces of the cells.

Both types of nerve fiber are present in nerves (Fig. 11d). In each nerve fiber, the axon appears as a central dot, surrounded by white space (which previously contained myelin, but has been lost during processing of the section).

If the neurons in the PNS are damaged, the axon distal to the site of the injury degenerates (Wallerian degeneration), and its myelin sheath also becomes fragmented. Schwann cells are stimulated to proliferate to repair the damage, and become phagocytic, engulfing these fragments, together with phagocytic white blood cells. The Schwann cells and connective tissue around the nerve form a scar. If the scar is not too great, the Schwann cells can bridge the scar, and the regenerating nerve can grow across this bridge and re-innervate their target organ.

In contrast, in the CNS (Chapter 10), the oligodendrocytes do not proliferate and they cannot repair any nerve damage.

Synapses

Most neurons synapse onto their target organs via a chemical synapse (Fig. 11f). At **chemical synapses**, a chemical neurotransmitter (e.g., acetylcholine, at neuromuscular junctions) is contained in synaptic vesicles in the terminal boutons of the nerve. When the nerve impulse reaches the terminal boutons, the vesicles release their contents into the narrow synaptic cleft between the synapse and the target organ. The neurotransmitter rapidly moves across the cleft, binds to receptors in the postsynaptic membrane of the target organ, and the target organ depolarizes.

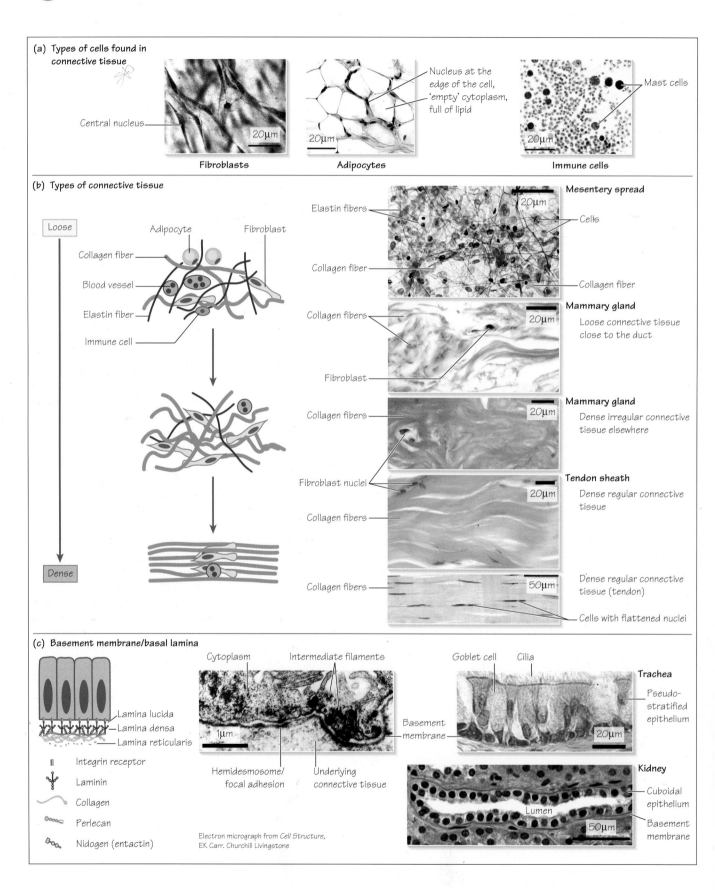

(a) Types of cells found in connective tissue

Central nucleus

20µm

Fibroblasts

Nucleus at the edge of the cell, 'empty' cytoplasm, full of lipid

20µm

Adipocytes

Mast cells

20µm

Immune cells

(b) Types of connective tissue

Loose

Adipocyte   Fibroblast

Collagen fiber

Blood vessel

Elastin fiber

Immune cell

Dense

Elastin fibers

Collagen fiber

Cells

Collagen fiber

20µm

Mesentery spread

Collagen fibers

Fibroblast

20µm

Mammary gland
Loose connective tissue close to the duct

Collagen fibers

20µm

Mammary gland
Dense irregular connective tissue elsewhere

Fibroblast nuclei

Collagen fibers

20µm

Tendon sheath
Dense regular connective tissue

Collagen fibers

50µm

Dense regular connective tissue (tendon)

Cells with flattened nuclei

(c) Basement membrane/basal lamina

Lamina lucida
Lamina densa
Lamina reticularis

Integrin receptor

Laminin

Collagen

Perlecan

Nidogen (entactin)

Cytoplasm   Intermediate filaments

1µm

Hemidesmosome/ focal adhesion

Underlying connective tissue

Basement membrane

Goblet cell   Cilia

Trachea
Pseudo-stratified epithelium

20µm

Kidney

Cuboidal epithelium

Lumen

Basement membrane

50µm

Electron micrograph from *Cell Structure,* EK Carr. Churchill Livingstone

Connective tissue lies under the epithelia of all tissues and organs. It provides both structural and metabolic support for the surrounding tissue, as it contains the blood vessels, and can also contain adipocytes. Adhesion of cells to the underlying connective tissue is essential for their survival. The extracellular matrix also regulates cell proliferation, migration, and differentiation.

Types of cell in connective tissue

• **Fibroblasts:** Fibroblasts (Fig. 12a) secrete the extracellular matrix that makes up the connective tissue.
• **Adipocytes:** These cells store fat. They usually look 'empty' in histology sections because lipid stored in these cells is extracted during the process of making the sections (Fig. 12a).
• **Immune cells:** These include macrophages, mast cells (Fig. 12a), and plasma cells.

Extracellular matrix in connective tissue

The extracellular matrix contains a mixture of proteoglycans, adhesive glycoproteins, and fibrous proteins.

Proteoglycans

• **Proteoglycans** contain repeating disaccharide units (glycosaminoglycans, or 'GAGs') bound to a protein core. (GAGs used to be known as 'ground substance'.) **GAGs** are highly negatively charged, hydrophilic, and heavily hydrated.
• There are four main groups of GAG: (1) hyaluronan (the simplest, which does not covalently link with proteins to form a proteoglycan); (2) chondroitin sulfate and dermatan sulfate; (3) heparan sulfate and heparin; (4) keratan sulfate.
• The large amount of water bound to GAGs gives connective tissue a high turgor, which means that it is good at resisting compressive forces.
• Proteoglycans are made by virtually all cells, and are secreted.

Adhesive glycoproteins

Adhesive glycoproteins are secreted extracellular proteins, which include various types of laminin and fibronectin. They bind to integrins in the cell membrane, and therefore help cells to adhere to the underlying extracellular matrix.

Fibrous proteins

Fibrous proteins include collagen and elastin (of which there are many types). Both collagen and elastin are secreted as precursor molecules (tropocollagen and tropoelastin). Mature elastic fibers consist of an inner core of cross-linked elastin and an outer coat of fibrillin (a glycoprotein). Collagen fibers consist of trimers, which can then assemble into higher-order structures.

The diversity of connective tissue arises from the variations in amount and type of components of the extracellular matrix.

Tendons, cartilage, and bone are specialized forms of extracellular matrix (see Chapters 15 and 16). In bone and teeth, the extracellular matrix becomes calcified.

Types of connective tissue

The organization of the extracellular matrix (Fig. 12b) varies from:
• **loose irregular** (where the numbers of cells and fibrous proteins are relatively low); to
• **dense irregular** (where there are more cells, and fibers); to
• **dense regular** (where the fibers are densely packed, and regularly arranged).

There is a continuous spectrum between these different types of connective tissue.

Basal lamina/basement membrane

The basal lamina is a specialized form of extracellular matrix. It consists of a thin layer, containing a dense meshwork of extracellular matrix proteins (laminin, type IV collagen, entactin, and proteoglycans, e.g., perlecan) (Fig. 12c). The specific content varies from tissue to tissue. These proteins bind to each other and form a highly dense, cross-linked extracellular matrix.

The cells in the epithelium are connected to the underlying basement membrane by integrins. Integrins are dimeric transmembrane proteins, which bind to laminin and fibronectin in the underlying basal lamina. Specialized integrins (bullous pemphigoid antigen (BPAG) 1 and 2, or α6β4 integrin) are found in hemidesmosomes. These are anchored to keratin (intermediate) filaments on the intracellular side of the plasma membrane.

The basement membrane is found:
• directly underneath epithelial cells;
• surrounding neuronal, muscle and fat cells;
• separating two sheets of cells, such as the endothelium of blood vessels and the epithelium of adjacent ducts in the kidney.

Connections between the cells and their underlying basement membrane are very important for their integrity and survival. For example, blistering skin diseases are caused by mutations in *BPAG1*. Muscular dystrophy is caused by mutations in the protein dystrophin in striated muscle. Dystrophin is involved in connecting the muscle cytoskeleton to the basal lamina.

The basal lamina is often difficult to see by light microscopy, unless it is thick or special stains are used, as shown here (Fig. 12c).

Electron microscopy (Fig. 12c) shows that it has three layers: **lamina lucida**, a clear layer between the cell and the underlying **lamina densa**, and the **lamina reticularis** (reticular lamina), which contains type III collagen or reticular fibers and is continuous with the underlying connective tissue).

13 Blood

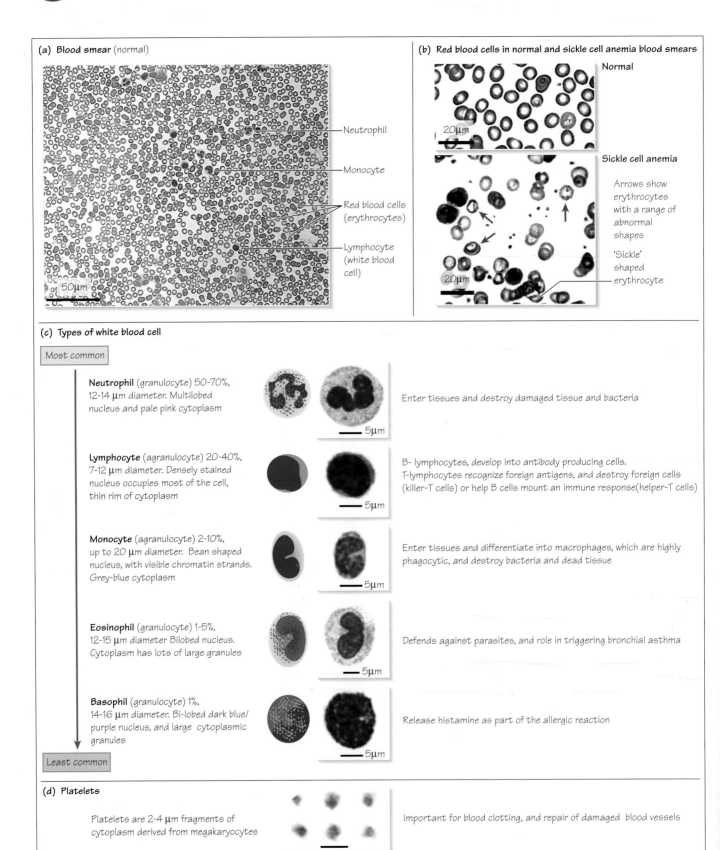

(a) Blood smear (normal)

Neutrophil

Monocyte

Red blood cells (erythrocytes)

Lymphocyte (white blood cell)

50μm

(b) Red blood cells in normal and sickle cell anemia blood smears

Normal

20μm

Sickle cell anemia

Arrows show erythrocytes with a range of abnormal shapes

'Sickle' shaped erythrocyte

20μm

(c) Types of white blood cell

Most common

Neutrophil (granulocyte) 50-70%, 12-14 μm diameter. Multilobed nucleus and pale pink cytoplasm

Enter tissues and destroy damaged tissue and bacteria

5μm

Lymphocyte (agranulocyte) 20-40%, 7-12 μm diameter. Densely stained nucleus occupies most of the cell, thin rim of cytoplasm

B- lymphocytes, develop into antibody producing cells. T-lymphocytes recognize foreign antigens, and destroy foreign cells (killer-T cells) or help B cells mount an immune response(helper-T cells)

5μm

Monocyte (agranulocyte) 2-10%, up to 20 μm diameter. Bean shaped nucleus, with visible chromatin strands. Grey-blue cytoplasm

Enter tissues and differentiate into macrophages, which are highly phagocytic, and destroy bacteria and dead tissue

5μm

Eosinophil (granulocyte) 1-5%, 12-15 μm diameter Bilobed nucleus. Cytoplasm has lots of large granules

Defends against parasites, and role in triggering bronchial asthma

5μm

Basophil (granulocyte) 1%, 14-16 μm diameter. Bi-lobed dark blue/purple nucleus, and large cytoplasmic granules

Release histamine as part of the allergic reaction

5μm

Least common

(d) Platelets

Platelets are 2-4 μm fragments of cytoplasm derived from megakaryocytes

Important for blood clotting, and repair of damaged blood vessels

5μm

Content and functions of blood

Blood transports gases, nutrients, waste, cells, and hormones throughout the body. It helps to regulate pH, temperature and water content of cells, protects against blood loss via clotting, and protects against disease through the actions of white blood cells and antibodies.

Blood consists of cells (~45%) and plasma (~55%). All the cells are made in the bone marrow.

The cells include red blood cells (erythrocytes: $\sim 5 \times 10^6$ per mL), white blood cells (leucocytes: $\sim 2 \times 10^3$ per mL), and platelets (thrombocytes: $\sim 2 \times 10^5$ per mL).

Blood plasma contains water (92%), proteins (such as hormones, serum albumin, and serum globulin), lipids (such as cholesterol), salts (such as urea), and glucose.

Red blood cells

Red blood cells (erythrocytes) are 'born' in the bone marrow, lose their nuclei, and become packed full of hemoglobin, which binds oxygen and carbon dioxide. These biconcave cells move through narrow capillaries more easily without a nucleus. Red blood cells are 7 μm in diameter, and are eosinophilic due to their high protein content (Fig. 13a).

In **sickle cell anemia**, red blood cells have abnormal shapes, including the characteristic 'sickle' cell shape due to mutations in hemoglobin (Fig. 13b). Cells are less deformable, and can get stuck in the capillaries, reducing blood flow, causing pain and organ damage.

The cells circulate for about 120 days, before disposal in the liver. About 3×10^6 erythrocytes die and are scavenged by the liver every second.

White blood cells

White blood cells are less common than red blood cells, as shown by a blood smear (Fig. 13a). There are five main type of white blood cell (leucocytes; Fig. 13c), which are divided into:
• **granulocytes** (neutrophils, eosinophils and basophils), which have a granular cytoplasm; and
• **agranulocytes** (lymphocytes and monocytes), which do not.

Granulocytes

Neutrophils (most common) contain a multilobed (2–5 lobes) nucleus, and contain azure (primary) granules (colored purple, due to sulfated glycoproteins that react with the stain), which secrete elastase and myeloperoxidase (antimicrobial enzymes), and paler (secondary) granules, which contain lysozyme and other proteases. They circulate for about 6–10 hours in the blood, and then enter tissues. They are motile and phagocytic, destroying damaged tissue and bacteria. After this activity, they self-destruct. They are important in inflammatory reactions.

Eosinophils (fairly rare in blood smears) have a bilobed nucleus. They are rare because they leave the blood system quickly after being manufactured in the bone marrow, entering the loose connective tissue in the respiratory and gastrointestinal tracts. They phagocytose antigen–antibody complexes. They also release histaminase and arylsulfatase B, which inactivates inflammatory reagents released by mast cells.

Basophils (very rare in blood smears) contain IgE receptors and are involved in immune responses to parasites. Granules in these cells contain histamine, prostaglandins, heparin, and serotinin, and are released in areas of damaged tissue. The released components increase blood flow to the area (inflammatory response). Histamine release also plays a role in allergic reactions.

Agranulocytes

Monocytes are the third most common white blood cells. They circulate in the blood for 1–3 days after birth, before migrating into body tissues, where they differentiate into phagocytic macrophages, and phagocytose dead cells and bacteria. They are important in the inflammatory response. They can also differentiate into osteoclasts, which are found in bone (see Chapter 16).

Monocytes (and macrophages), neutrophils, eosinophils, basophils (and mast cells) are all derived from a common **myeloid** progenitor in the bone marrow.

Lymphocytes are the second most common white blood cell. There are two kinds, B-cells and T-cells, both of which are born in the bone marrow. They are both derived from a common lymphoid progenitor cell.

B-lymphocytes mature in the bone marrow. They are involved in the humoral antibody response: B-cells and their progeny develop into **plasma** cells, which manufacture and secrete antibodies. They are important in mounting an immune response to infectious bacteria.

Multiple myeloma (a type of blood cancer) develops when plasma cells become transformed and divide in an uncontrolled way.

T-lymphocytes mature in the thymus. They do not make antibodies, and the antigen receptors on their surfaces are different to those on B-cells.

The different types of T-cell and B-cell cannot be distinguished using histological stains, but can be distinguished using immunostaining for the different cell surface markers that these cells express.

Other immune cells

• **Dendritic and reticular cells:** present antigens to lymphocytes on their cell surface.
• **Mast cells:** bone marrow-derived cells involved in allergic reactions. They have receptors for IgE antibodies on its surface, and release histamine, heparin, etc.

Platelets

These are cytoplasmic fragments formed by multinucleated cells (**megakaryocytes**; see Chapter 14) in the bone marrow (Fig. 13d). They adhere to collagenous tissue at the edges of wounds to form plugs, promote the formation of clots, and secrete factors involved in vascular repair. They do not have a nucleus, but contain mitochondria, microtubules, actin filaments, glycogen granules, some Golgi, and ribosomes.

Red blood cells and platelets are derived from a common myeloid progenitor.

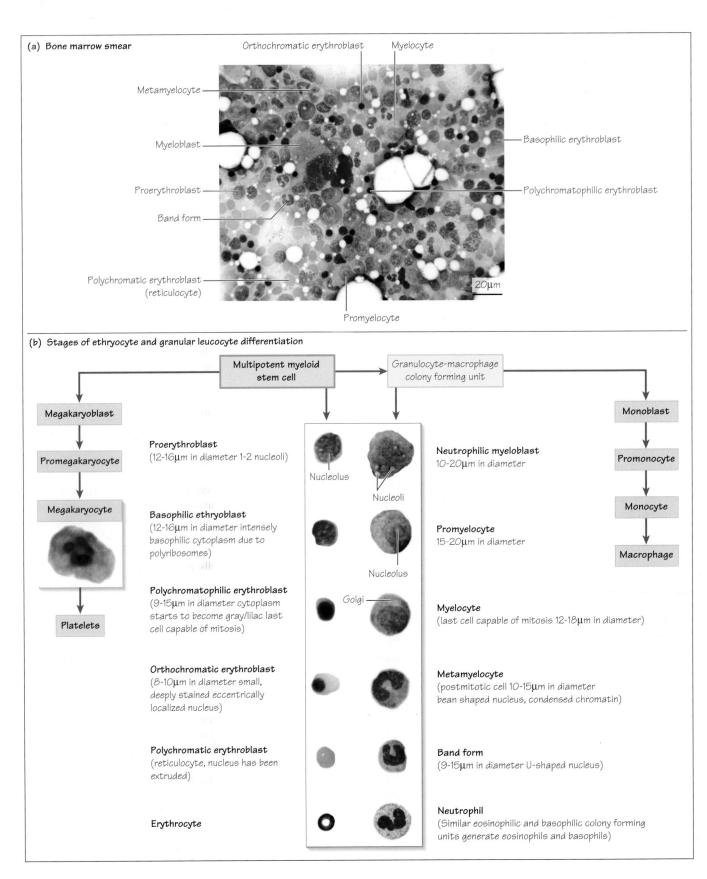

(a) Bone marrow smear

Orthochromatic erythroblast

Myelocyte

Metamyelocyte

Myeloblast

Proerythroblast

Band form

Polychromatic erythroblast (reticulocyte)

Basophilic erythroblast

Polychromatophilic erythroblast

Promyelocyte

20μm

(b) Stages of ethryocyte and granular leucocyte differentiation

Multipotent myeloid stem cell

Granulocyte-macrophage colony forming unit

Megakaryoblast

Promegakaryocyte

Megakaryocyte

Platelets

Monoblast

Promonocyte

Monocyte

Macrophage

Proerythroblast
(12-16μm in diameter 1-2 nucleoli)

Nucleolus

Nucleoli

Basophilic ethryoblast
(12-16μm in diameter intensely basophilic cytoplasm due to polyribosomes)

Polychromatophilic erythroblast
(9-15μm in diameter cytoplasm starts to become gray/lilac last cell capable of mitosis)

Golgi

Nucleolus

Orthochromatic erythroblast
(8-10μm in diameter small, deeply stained eccentrically localized nucleus)

Polychromatic erythroblast
(reticulocyte, nucleus has been extruded)

Erythrocyte

Neutrophilic myeloblast
10-20μm in diameter

Promyelocyte
15-20μm in diameter

Myelocyte
(last cell capable of mitosis 12-18μm in diameter)

Metamyelocyte
(postmitotic cell 10-15μm in diameter bean shaped nucleus, condensed chromatin)

Band form
(9-15μm in diameter U-shaped nucleus)

Neutrophil
(Similar eosinophilic and basophilic colony forming units generate eosinophils and basophils)

Hemopoiesis is the process by which mature blood cells develop from precursor cells. It occurs continuously throughout embryonic and adult life, as new blood cells constantly replace old mature blood cells in the circulation.

Erythrocytes, granulocytes (neutrophils, eosinophils, and basophils), agranulocytes (lymphocytes and monocytes), and platelets are all formed in the bone marrow (Fig. 14a), which are found in the spaces between trabeculae in spongy bone.

The bone marrow contains **pluripotent stem cells** that differentiate into **multipotent lymphoid stem cells** and **multipotent myeloid stem cells**.

Multipotent lymphoid stem cells

These cells further differentiate into T- and B-**lymphocytes** (also known as T- and B-cells).

B-lymphocytes can develop into antibody-secreting **plasma** cells in lymphoid tissue.

B-cells mature in the bone marrow, start to express immunoglobulins on their surface (IgM and IgD), and are presented with 'self-antigens' to test their binding specificity. If they pass this test, and do not react with 'self-antigens', they leave the bone marrow and travel via the bloodstream to the lymph nodes and other lymphoid tissue.

T-cells mature in the thymus, by interacting with thymic epithelial cells (see Chapter 42). They then travel, via the bloodstream, to peripheral lymphoid tissue. Antigens are presented to T-cells via antigen-presenting cells in these tissues. T-cells can further differentiate into helper T-cells (CD4+) and cytotoxic T-cells (CD8+). CD4 and CD8 are types of 'cluster of differentiation' glycoproteins found on the cell surface.

Multipotent myeloid stem cells

These cells further differentiate (Fig. 14b), as follows.

Megakaryocyte colony-forming units

These develop into megakaryocytes, which form platelets. Megakaryocytes can be identified in the bone marrow as huge cells (up to 150 μm in diameter), which are multinucleated.

Erythroid colony-forming units

These cells differentiate into erythroblasts, and finally into erythrocytes (red blood cells). During differentiation, the cells gradually shrink from 12–16 μm in diameter, and finally, the nucleus is lost at the reticulocyte (polychromatic erythroblast) stage. Reticulocytes are released into the bloodstream, and mature into red blood cells within 24 hours.

Granulocyte/neutrophil colony-forming units

These differentiate into monocytes and neutrophils.
• **Monocytes** subsequently develop into macrophages.
• **Neutrophils** (Fig. 14b) develop via a number of immature stages. For example, myelocytes are an intermediate stage in neutrophil formation, and are the last stage at which this type of cell can undergo cell division.

Basophil colony-forming units

These generate basophils, via a number of stages, which appear similar to those of the neutrophil colony-forming units, except that the cells are basophilic. Basophils can develop further to form mast cells.

Eosinophil colony-forming units

These generate eosinophils, via a number of stages, which appear similar to those of the neutrophil colony-forming units, except that the cells are eosinophilic.

In general, precursor cells in the bone marrow are larger in diameter than mature red and white blood cells.

Blood disorders

Various leukemias can result from the abnormal proliferation of precursor white (or red) blood cells, as follows.

Chronic lymphocytic leukemia

Chronic lymphocytic leukemia (CLL) is the most common form of leukemia (about 25% of all diagnosed cases) and mainly affects adults. The cells causing this disease are B-cells, which have not fully differentiated, but resemble fully mature B-lymphocytes. The increase in these immature B-lymphocytes can cause patients to become immunocompromised. This disease can be diagnosed from a blood smear. Normal blood smears do not normally contain more than 2.5×10^9 lymphocytes per liter. In CLL, this number can increase more than 4-fold to over 10×10^9 cells per liter (this is called lymphocytosis).

Acute lymphoblastic leukemia

This form of leukemia is most common in children (two-thirds of cases) and is a malignant disorder of lymphoblastic cells.

Acute myeloid leukemia

Acute myeloid leukemia (AML) results from proliferation of myeloid stem cells in the bone marrow, and is the most common malignant myeloid disorder in adults. It is a heterogeneous disorder, affecting any of the blast cell stages in hemopoiesis. It can be diagnosed from bone marrow smears, which are examined for abnormal levels of myeloblasts. (The numbers increase such that more than 30% of all the cells in the bone marrow will be immature white blood cell types.) AML commonly causes death as a result of bone marrow failure.

Aplastic anemia

This is a rare hemopoietic blood cell disorder, commonly caused by the destruction of bone marrow stem cells by reactive lymphocytes. It results in a reduction of all blood cells (white, red, and platelets). There is a range of other anemias including:
• **microcytic anemia** (red blood cells smaller than normal), commonly caused by lack of iron;
• **macrocytic anemia** (red blood cells larger than normal), commonly caused by a deficiency of vitamin B12 or folic acid;
• **hemolytic anemia**, results from an abnormal breakdown of red blood cells.

15 Cartilage

(a) Cartilage organization

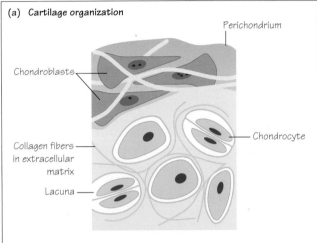

Perichondrium

Chondroblasts

Chondrocyte

Collagen fibers in extracellular matrix

Lacuna

(b) Hyaline cartilage in fetal foot

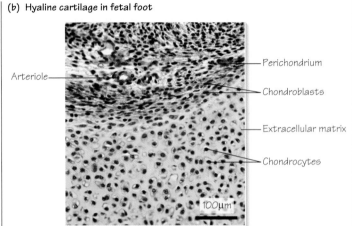

Arteriole

Perichondrium

Chondroblasts

Extracellular matrix

Chondrocytes

100μm

(c) Hyaline cartilage (epiphyseal plate)

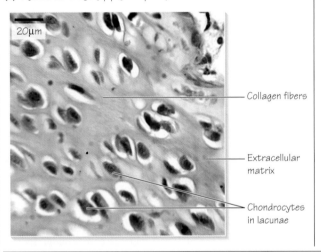

20μm

Collagen fibers

Extracellular matrix

Chondrocytes in lacunae

(d) Hyaline cartilage in the trachea (trichrome stain)

Extracellular matrix

Chondrocytes

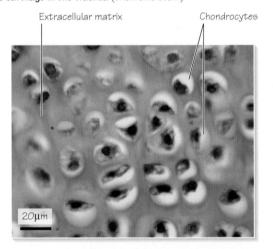

20μm

(e) Elastic cartilage (epiglottis)

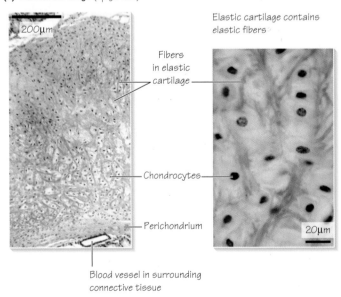

200μm

Elastic cartilage contains elastic fibers

Fibers in elastic cartilage

Chondrocytes

Perichondrium

Blood vessel in surrounding connective tissue

20μm

(f) Fibrocartilage (invertebral disc)

Chondrocytes in lacuna

Collagen fibers

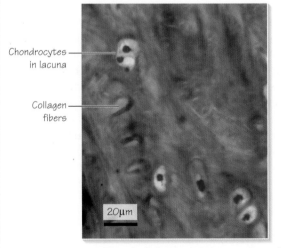

20μm

Fibrocartilage does not have a perichondrium. It is very rich in collagen fibers, and there is less matrix material around the chondrocytes than in hyaline cartilage

Cartilage is a rigid form of connective tissue. It consists of cells embedded in an extracellular matrix, the content of which defines their property. The extracellular matrix is a mixture of glycosaminoglycans (GAGs), fibers and structural glycoproteins (see Chapter 12).

Cartilage is thin, does not have a blood supply (avascular), is flexible, resistant to compressive forces, and yet can bend.

Functions of cartilage
1 A supporting framework for the walls of airways in the nose, trachea, larynx and bronchi, preventing airway collapse.
2 Forms the articulating surfaces of bones.
3 Forms the template for the growth and development of most of the fetal skeleton including long bones. In children, the cartilaginous epiphyseal growth plates at the ends of long bones show up on X-rays. They disappear when adults reach their full height.

Constituents of cartilage
Cells
The cells in cartilage are **chondroblasts** and **chondrocytes** (*chondro* means 'cartilage'). Chondroblasts are found in the outer covering layer of cartilage (Fig. 15a). They secrete the extracellular matrix and fibers and, as they do so, they become trapped inside it and mature into chondrocytes.

In **growing cartilage**, the chondrocytes can divide, and the daughter cells remain close together in groups, forming a 'nest' of 2–4 cells. These trapped cells sit together in clear areas called **lacunae** (*lacunae* means 'little lakes').

Active chondrocytes are large secretory cells with a basophilic (purple staining) cytoplasm, which arises from a high content of rough endoplasmic reticulum (ER).

Older chondrocytes contain fat droplets.

Fixation of cartilage usually causes some shrinkage between the cell border and the lacunar wall, so that the lacunae look more prominent in fixed tissue.

Extracellular matrix
The extracellular matrix (ECM) of cartilage is made up of **aggrecan** (10%), water (75%) and fibers. **Aggrecan** is formed of aggregates of up to 100 molecules of the GAG, chondroitin sulfate, bound to hyaluronic acid. Chondroitin sulfate is rubbery, provides cartilage with resilience, and this type of GAG is only found in cartilage.

Fibers in cartilage are either collagen, or a mixture of collagen and elastin fibers. A network of collagen fibers generates a very high tensile strength. Elastic fibers provide elasticity.

A layer of dense irregular connective tissue called the **perichondrium** (*peri* means 'around') surrounds hyaline and elastic cartilage. The outer layer of the perichondrium contains collagen-producing fibroblasts, and the inner layer contains chondroblasts.

Unlike other connective tissue, cartilage is **avascular** (like epithelium). Cartilage is nourished by long-range diffusion from nearby capillaries in the perichondrium. Therefore, cartilage can never become very thick, as diffusion would not be sufficient to supply the cartilage with nutrients and oxygen.

Two ways that cartilage grows
- **Interstitial growth:** chondrocytes grow and divide and lay down more matrix inside the existing cartilage. This mainly occurs during childhood and adolescence.
- **Appositional growth:** new surface layers of matrix are added to the pre-existing matrix by new chondroblasts from the perichondrium.

Types of cartilage
There are three types of cartilage: hyaline, elastic, and fibro-cartilage.

Hyaline cartilage
This is the most common, and the weakest type of cartilage. Its name comes from the glassy appearance of living cartilage (*hyalos* is Greek for 'glass').
- It stains light purple (basophilic) in H&E.
- It contains dispersed fine type II collagen fibers, which provide strength. (These are difficult to see in sections.)
- It has an outer layer called the perichondrium.
- Hyaline cartilage is a precursor of bone (Fig. 15b).
- Hyaline cartilage is found in epiphyseal growth plates (Fig. 15c), ribs, nose, larynx,and trachea (Fig. 15d).

Elastic cartilage
- It is found in the external ear, larynx, and epiglottis (Fig. 15e), where it helps to maintain their shapes.
- It is flexible and resilient and contains elastic as well as collagen fibers.
- The chondrocytes are found in a threadlike network of **elastic fibers** within the matrix.
- It has a perichondrium.

Fibro-cartilage
- Fibro-cartilage is found in joint capsules, ligaments, tendon insertions, and intervertebral discs (Fig. 15f).
- It is made up of alternating layers of hyaline cartilage matrix and thick layers of dense parallel bundles of collagen fibers, oriented in the direction of applied stresses, to reinforce this cartilage.
- This is strongest kind of cartilage.
- It does not have a perichondrium as it is usually sandwiched between hyaline cartilage and tendons or ligaments.

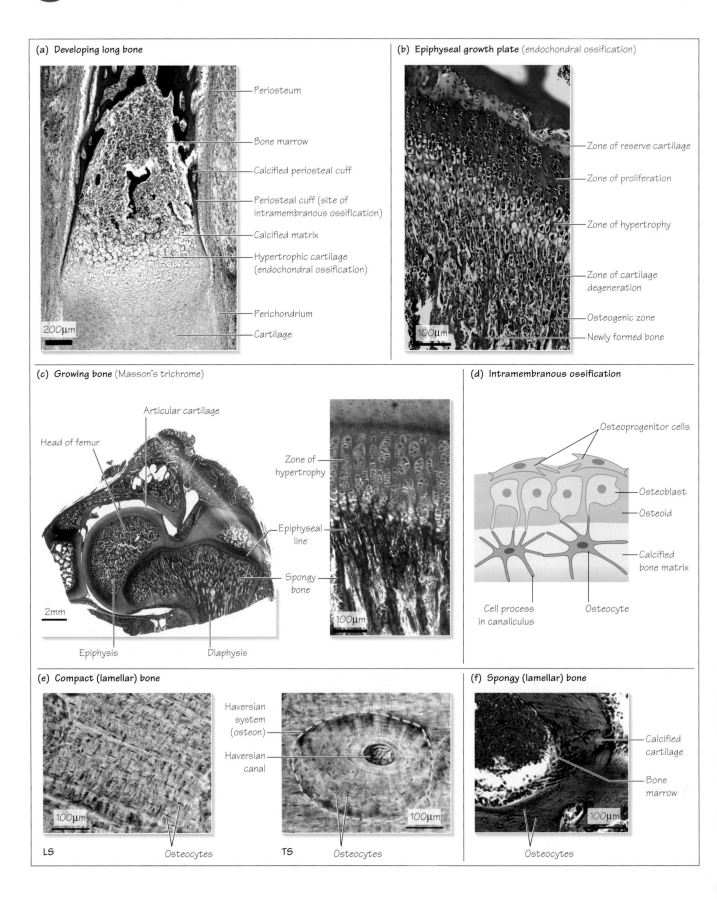

(a) Developing long bone

- Periosteum
- Bone marrow
- Calcified periosteal cuff
- Periosteal cuff (site of intramembranous ossification)
- Calcified matrix
- Hypertrophic cartilage (endochondral ossification)
- Perichondrium
- Cartilage

200μm

(b) Epiphyseal growth plate (endochondral ossification)

- Zone of reserve cartilage
- Zone of proliferation
- Zone of hypertrophy
- Zone of cartilage degeneration
- Osteogenic zone
- Newly formed bone

100μm

(c) Growing bone (Masson's trichrome)

- Articular cartilage
- Head of femur
- Epiphysis
- Diaphysis
- Zone of hypertrophy
- Epiphyseal line
- Spongy bone

2mm

100μm

(d) Intramembranous ossification

- Osteoprogenitor cells
- Osteoblast
- Osteoid
- Calcified bone matrix
- Osteocyte
- Cell process in canaliculus

(e) Compact (lamellar) bone

- Haversian system (osteon)
- Haversian canal

100μm

LS — Osteocytes

TS — Osteocytes

100μm

(f) Spongy (lamellar) bone

- Calcified cartilage
- Bone marrow

100μm

Osteocytes

Bone, like cartilage, is a strong, flexible and semi-rigid form of connective tissue. It can withstand compression forces, and resists bending, twisting, compression and stretch.

It contains cells embedded in an extracellular calcified collagen rich matrix, which makes bone very strong.

Unlike cartilage, it is highly vascularized.

Functions of bone

1 Support: Bones provide a structural framework for the body.
2 Protection: Bones in the skull and the ribs protect internal organs such as the brain, and the heart and lungs, respectively.
3 Assisting movement: Bones provide the major attachment sites for muscles, and joints between bones allow movement to take place.
4 Mineral homeostasis: Bone stores calcium and phosphorus.
5 Blood cell production: Cells are produced in the bone marrow.

Types of bone formation

1 Endochondral (most common): bone forms on a temporary cartilage model (Fig. 16a–c).
• Cartilage grows (zone of proliferation), the chondrocytes mature (zone of maturation) and start to hypertrophy (zone of hypertrophy).
• The matrix starts to calcify, and the chondrocytes die (zone of cartilage degeneration).
• The fragmented calcified matrix left behind acts as structural framework for bony material. Osteoprogenitor cells and blood vessels from the periosteum invade this area, proliferate, and differentiate into osteoblasts, which start to lay down bone matrix (osteogenic zone).
2 Intramembranous (rarer): bone forms directly onto fibrous connective tissue (the periosteal cuff) without an intermediate cartilage stage (Fig. 16a,d). Intramembranous ossification occurs in a few specialized places such as the flat bones of skull (i.e. parietal bone), mandible, maxilla, and clavicles.

Bone formation in the fetus

The primary ossification center forms first in the **diaphysis** (shaft) of long bones. Later on a secondary ossification center forms in the **epiphysis** (rounded end of long bones).

Bone replaces cartilage in the epiphysis and diaphysis, except in the epiphyseal plate region (Fig. 16b,c). Here the bone continues to grow, until maturity (around 18 years old). The growth plate can be seen in X-rays.

The long shafts of bone are made up of a thick walled cylinder that encloses a central bone marrow cavity.

Content of bone

Cells

Osteoprogenitor cells, osteoblasts, osteocytes, and osteoclasts are all found in bone.

Osteoprogenitor cells are the 'stem' cells of bone, and are the source of new **osteoblasts**.

Osteoblasts line the surface of bone, and secrete collagen and the organic matrix of bone (osteoid), which then becomes calcified.

Osteoblasts become trapped in the organic matrix, and differentiate into **osteocytes.**

Osteocytes maintain bone tissue. They sit in the calcified matrix, in small spaces called lacunae (singular, lacuna). They project fine processes out through small channels (canaliculi), which transport nutrients and waste. The tips of these processes contact those from other osteocytes, and are connected by communicating gap junctions.

Osteoclasts are large, multinucleated (4–6 nuclei) cells with a 'ruffled border', that resorb bone matrix, and are important for bone remodeling, growth, and repair. They secrete enzymes (e.g., carbonic anhydrase), to acidify and decalcify the matrix, and hydrolases, to break down the matrix once it is decalcified.

They are **not** derived from osteoprogenitor cells, but are derived from monocytes/macrophages (see Chapter 13).

Bone is remodeled in response to mechanical stress and hormones (parathyroid hormone stimulates resorption and calcitonin inhibits resorption).

Extracellular matrix

The extracellular matrix (ECM) (30%) contains proteoglycans: glycosaminoglycans, osteonectin (anchors bone mineral to collagen), glycoproteins, and osteocalcin (calcium-binding protein).

Fibers

Bone contains collagen fibers (90% are type I fibers), which help to resist tensile stresses.

Bone also contains **water** (25%) and **hydroxyapatite**, a bone mineral (~70% of bone).

Bone is hard because the ECM is calcified. Calcium salts crystallize in the spaces between collagen fibers.

The **periosteum** is a dense fibrous layer, found on the outside of bone where muscles insert, but not in regions of bone covered by articular cartilage. It contains bone-forming (osteoprogenitor) cells.

The **endosteum** lines the inner surfaces of bones.

Types of bone

Woven (primary) bone is the first type of bone to be formed at any site, and contains randomly arranged collagen fibers. This is quickly replaced by **lamellar** bone, in which collagen fibers become remodeled into parallel layers.

There are two types of **mature bone**, compact (80% of all bone) and spongy (20%).

Compact bone

Compact bone is found in the shafts (diaphyses) of long bones (Fig. 16e). Older compact bone is organized into **Haversian systems** (or **osteons**). The osteocytes are arranged in concentric rings of bone matrix called lamellae (little plates), around a central Haversian canal (which runs longitudinally), and their processes run in interconnecting canaliculi. The central Haversian canal, and horizontal canals (perforating or Volkmann's canals) contain blood vessels and nerves from the periosteum.

Spongy (cancellous) bone

Cancellous bone is found at the **ends of long bones** (in the epiphysis, Fig. 16c,f). It contains red bone marrow in large open spaces (marrow spaces) between a network of bony plates (trabeculae).

Growth and nourishment of bone

Bone is well vascularized. The central cavity contains blood vessels and stores bone marrow. All osteocytes in bone are within 0.2 mm of a capillary.

17 Heart

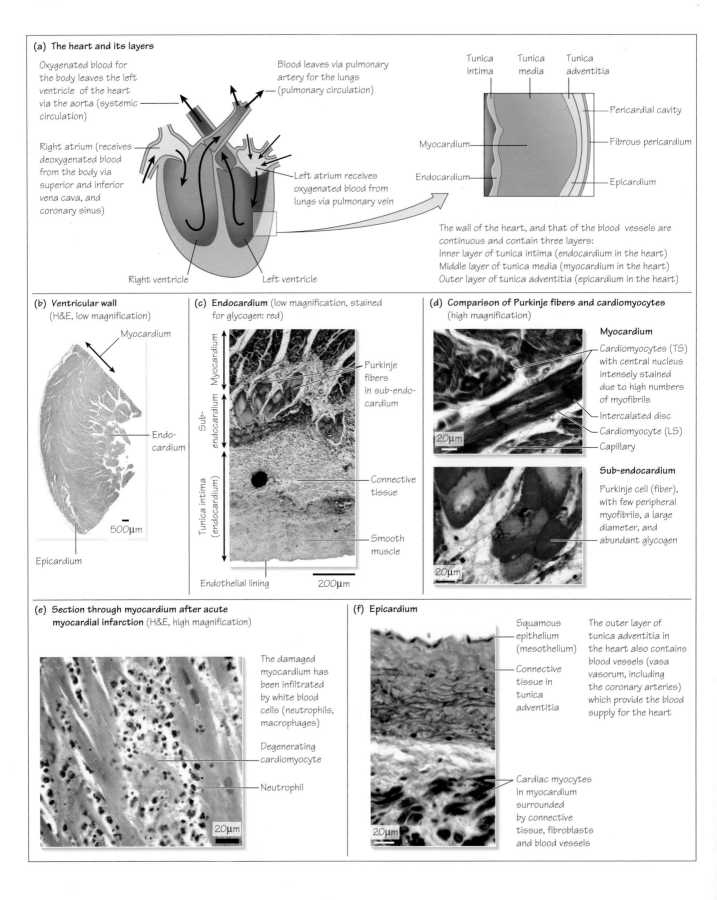

(a) The heart and its layers

Oxygenated blood for the body leaves the left ventricle of the heart via the aorta (systemic circulation)

Blood leaves via pulmonary artery for the lungs (pulmonary circulation)

Right atrium (receives deoxygenated blood from the body via superior and inferior vena cava, and coronary sinus)

Left atrium receives oxygenated blood from lungs via pulmonary vein

Right ventricle

Left ventricle

Tunica intima

Tunica media

Tunica adventitia

Myocardium

Endocardium

Pericardial cavity

Fibrous pericardium

Epicardium

The wall of the heart, and that of the blood vessels are continuous and contain three layers:
Inner layer of tunica intima (endocardium in the heart)
Middle layer of tunica media (myocardium in the heart)
Outer layer of tunica adventitia (epicardium in the heart)

(b) Ventricular wall (H&E, low magnification)

Myocardium

Endo-cardium

Epicardium

500μm

(c) Endocardium (low magnification, stained for glycogen: red)

Myocardium

Sub-endocardium

Tunica intima (endocardium)

Purkinje fibers in sub-endo-cardium

Connective tissue

Smooth muscle

Endothelial lining

200μm

(d) Comparison of Purkinje fibers and cardiomyocytes (high magnification)

Myocardium

Cardiomyocytes (TS) with central nucleus intensely stained due to high numbers of myofibrils

Intercalated disc

Cardiomyocyte (LS)

Capillary

20μm

Sub-endocardium

Purkinje cell (fiber), with few peripheral myofibrils, a large diameter, and abundant glycogen

20μm

(e) Section through myocardium after acute myocardial infarction (H&E, high magnification)

The damaged myocardium has been infiltrated by white blood cells (neutrophils, macrophages)

Degenerating cardiomyocyte

Neutrophil

20μm

(f) Epicardium

Squamous epithelium (mesothelium)

Connective tissue in tunica adventitia

The outer layer of tunica adventitia in the heart also contains blood vessels (vasa vasorum, including the coronary arteries) which provide the blood supply for the heart

Cardiac myocytes in myocardium surrounded by connective tissue, fibroblasts and blood vessels

20μm

 Histology at a Glance, 1st edition. © Michelle Peckham. Published 2011 by Blackwell Publishing Ltd.

The heart is part of the cardiovascular system.

This system is important for:
• pumping blood around the body (systemic circulation) and between the heart and the lungs (pulmonary circulation);
• distributing oxygen, nutrients, hormones, and immune cells around the body;
• removing carbon dioxide and metabolic waste;
• regulating temperature.

Throughout the body, the walls of the heart and the blood vessels (or tubes) that make up the cardiovascular system contain three layers (Fig. 17a):
• **tunica intima**: inner layer that consists of flat endothelial cells supported by a basement membrane and delicate collagenous tissue;
• **tunica media**: intermediate muscular layer;
• **tunica adventitia**: outer supporting tissue layer (sometimes called tunica externa).

The muscular walls of the cardiovascular system only have one layer of muscle, in contrast to two or even three layers of muscle in the gut.

The three layers of the heart (tunica intima, tunica media, and tunica externa) are called the **endocardium**, **myocardium**, and **epicardium**, respectively (Fig. 17b).

Tunica intima/endocardium

The endocardium consists of a simple squamous epithelium (endothelium), which lines the endocardium, and underlying layers of connective tissue, in which the middle layer contains smooth muscle cells.

The innermost connective tissue layer is called the **subendocardium** (Fig. 17c). This layer contains the cells specialized for conduction: Purkinje cells (see below).

The lining epithelial layer is continuous with the epithelium lining all the blood vessels in the circulatory system.

Purkinje fibers are cardiac muscle fibers that are specialized for conduction. They are found in the subendocardium of the ventricles (a connective tissue layer). Purkinje cells differ from normal cardiac cells (Fig. 17d) in the following ways.
• Purkinje fibers do not contain many myofibrils, and those present are found at the cell periphery, which is demonstrated here by the less intense staining compared to cardiac muscle.
• They have higher levels of glycogen than cardiomyocytes.
• There are no intercalated discs between the cells, but desmosomes and gap junctions are present and connect these cells to each other.

• Purkinje fibers are larger than cardiac muscle cells, and do not have T-tubules.

The heart is stimulated to contract rhythmically by impulses generated by the sino-atrial (S-A) node. Impulses from the S-A node are conducted via the internodal pathway to the atrio-ventricular (A-V) node, and then into the ventricles. The left and right bundles of Purkinje fibers are responsible for the spread of the impulse around the ventricles.

Tunica media/myocardium

This 'middle' layer of the heart is called the myocardium.

The myocardium contains cardiac muscle cells (cardiomyocytes), blood vessels, fibroblasts, and small amounts of connective tissue.

Intercalated discs connect the cardiomyocytes to each other (see Chapter 9 and Fig. 17d). Importantly, gap junctions in the intercalated discs are responsible for communication between cardiomyocytes and the spread of electrical conduction around the heart.

The striated appearance of the cardiomyocytes is due to the regular arrangement of muscle sarcomeres in myofibrils that are packed into these cells (see Chapter 9).

A high-magnification image of the myocardium, taken from a patient who has had a heart attack (acute myocardial infarction; Fig. 17e), shows how the cardiomyocytes have become damaged. The tissue around the cardiomyocytes is full of white blood cells (mainly neutrophils and macrophages) that have escaped from the blood vessels, and which are engulfing the damaged tissue.

Tunica adventitia/epicardium

This outermost layer of the heart is called the epicardium (Fig. 17f).

The epicardium consists of a layer of flattened (squamous) epithelial cells and underlying connective tissue.

This layer of epithelium is called the **mesothelium**, as it lines the closed pericardial cavity which surrounds the heart. The mesothelium secretes fluid into the pericardial cavity, which lubricates the movements of the epicardium on the pericardium.

The epicardium contains coronary arteries, veins, vasa vasorum, connective tissue, and autonomic nerves that supply the myocardium.

Vasa vasorum are small blood vessels that supply the heart and the larger blood vessels, such as the aorta.

18 Arteries and arterioles

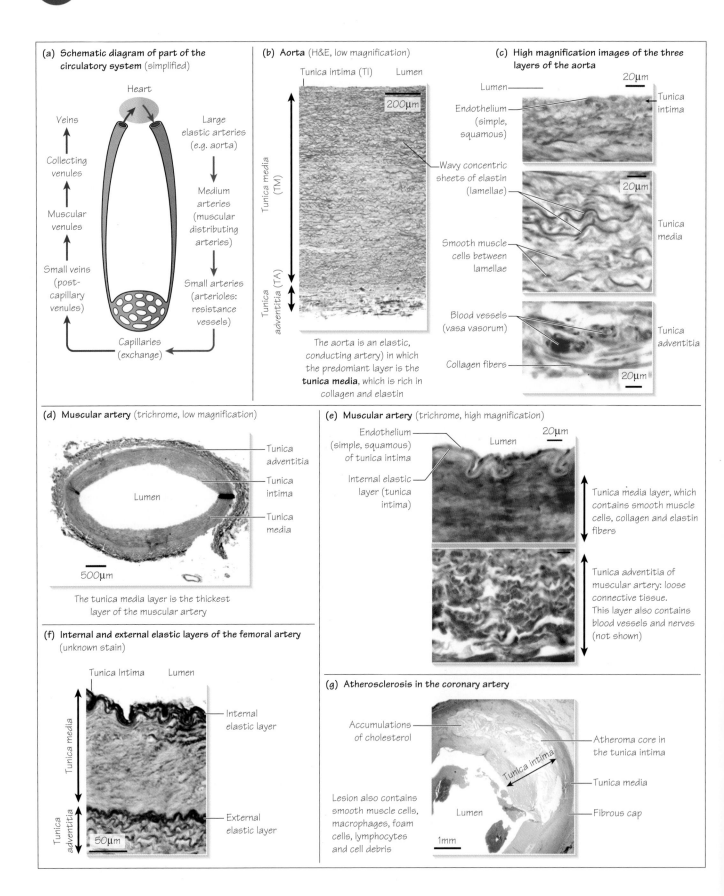

(a) Schematic diagram of part of the circulatory system (simplified)

Heart

Veins

Collecting venules

Muscular venules

Small veins (post-capillary venules)

Capillaries (exchange)

Large elastic arteries (e.g. aorta)

Medium arteries (muscular distributing arteries)

Small arteries (arterioles: resistance vessels)

(b) Aorta (H&E, low magnification)

Tunica intima (TI)   Lumen

200µm

Tunica media (TM)

Tunica adventitia (TA)

The aorta is an elastic, conducting artery) in which the predomiant layer is the **tunica media**, which is rich in collagen and elastin

(c) High magnification images of the three layers of the aorta

20µm

Lumen

Endothelium (simple, squamous)

Tunica intima

Wavy concentric sheets of elastin (lamellae)

20µm

Smooth muscle cells between lamellae

Tunica media

Blood vessels (vasa vasorum)

Collagen fibers

Tunica adventitia

20µm

(d) Muscular artery (trichrome, low magnification)

Tunica adventitia

Tunica intima

Tunica media

Lumen

500µm

The tunica media layer is the thickest layer of the muscular artery

(f) Internal and external elastic layers of the femoral artery (unknown stain)

Tunica Intima   Lumen

Tunica media

Tunica adventitia

Internal elastic layer

External elastic layer

50µm

(e) Muscular artery (trichrome, high magnification)

Endothelium (simple, squamous) of tunica intima

Internal elastic layer (tunica intima)

Lumen

20µm

Tunica media layer, which contains smooth muscle cells, collagen and elastin fibers

Tunica adventitia of muscular artery: loose connective tissue. This layer also contains blood vessels and nerves (not shown)

(g) Atherosclerosis in the coronary artery

Accumulations of cholesterol

Atheroma core in the tunica intima

Tunica intima

Tunica media

Lumen

Fibrous cap

Lesion also contains smooth muscle cells, macrophages, foam cells, lymphocytes and cell debris

1mm

In the systemic circulation, oxygenated blood (shown as red in Fig. 18a) leaves the heart and is pumped around the body through a series of blood vessels.

Blood leaving the heart enters large elastic 'conducting' arteries, which conduct the flow of blood from the heart into smaller arteries.

Blood then flows into distributing (**muscular**) arteries. These are about the size of a pencil in diameter, and are all named (e.g., femoral artery, brachial artery). The blood is distributed into smaller arteries (**arterioles**) before entering the **capillaries**. (See Chapter 19 and Fig. 19a,b for more on small arteries and arterioles.)

Capillaries are small, thin-walled structures that allow the transport of gases and nutrients between the lumen of the blood vessel and the surrounding tissues. Deoxygenated blood (blue, Fig. 18a) flows out of capillaries into small veins (**venules**), into medium veins and then into large veins before being returned to the heart.

The structure of blood vessels varies throughout the body, mainly by variations in the middle (**tunica media**) layer, and these variations in structure are important for their functions.

Elastic arteries

The elastic arteries (Fig. 18b) receive blood directly from the heart under high pressure. They include the aorta and its largest branches (the common carotid, brachiocephalic, subclavian, and common iliac arteries). These arteries have a diameter greater than 1 cm.

The walls of these arteries need to be able to accommodate the large changes in blood pressure between systole and diastole. When blood is pumped into the arteries during systole, the wall of the artery distends. Collagenous fibers in the tunica media and adventitia layers prevent a large distension.

During diastole (the relaxation phase of the cardiac cycle), blood pressure is maintained by the elastic recoil of the arteries in diastole, which forces blood away from the heart and into the rest of the circulation. The elastic recoil also forces blood back towards the heart, but this blood is prevented from re-entering the heart by the closure of the aortic and pulmonary valves.

The **tunica intima** (Fig. 18c) consists of:
• a simple squamous lining layer of cells (**endothelium**) which is continuous with the endothelium of the heart. This layer is important for forming a selective permeability barrier between the tissues and the blood;
• a **basement membrane**;
• a thin layer of **loose connective tissue** containing elastin and collagen fibers, and contractile smooth muscle cells;
• an **internal elastic layer**, which is continuous with the underlying elastic layer in the tunica media.

The lining endothelial cells can become 'activated' in response to external stimuli, and this can lead to vascular diseases such as atherosclerosis.

The **tunica media** (**middle layer,** Fig. 18c) is the most prominent layer. It contains:

• concentric sheets (lamellae) of elastin fibers, and collagen fibers. There are gaps (fenestrations) in these sheets, to allow diffusion of substances within this layer. Adults have about 40–70 lamellae, and the number can increase in hypertension;
• smooth muscle cells (myointimal cells), which synthesize the collagen and elastin in the tunica media layer, and lie between the sheets of elastin.

The **tunica adventitia** (Fig. 18b,c) is a thin outer layer. It contains:
• connective tissue (collagen and elastin);
• fibroblasts and macrophages; and
• small blood vessels (**vasa vasorum**) and nerves.

The vasa vasorum provide the outer regions of these large arteries with nutrients. The inner region is supplied by nutrients from the lumen of the artery. Small arteries do not require vasa vasorum.

Muscular arteries

These are the 'distributing' arteries. They have a large diameter of 2–10 mm. While they are smaller than elastic arteries, they are mostly large enough that they are all named (e.g., brachial artery, femoral artery, coronary artery).

They contain a prominent layer of smooth muscle in the tunica media (Fig. 18d–f) and a regular lumen, distinguishing them from muscular veins (Chapter 19).

The **tunica intima** (Fig. 18e) consists of:
• a single outer layer of flattened endothelial cells;
• an underlying basement membrane and subendothelial connective tissue;
• a inner layer of elastic fibers (the inner elastic layer; IEL).

The **tunica media** (Fig. 18e) is the most prominent layer. It consists of:
• a thick layer of smooth muscle cells, arranged circumferentially around the lumen of the artery, and embedded in an elastic matrix.
• an external elastic layer (EEL), the outermost layer of the tunica media (Fig. 18f).

The smooth muscle cells run circumferentially, and can contract (squeeze, or constrict) to reduce the size of the lumen, or relax, to increase (dilate) the size of the lumen. This changes the amount of blood that is allowed to flow through these arteries.

The **tunica adventitia** (Fig. 18e) is fairly broad. It contains:
• collagen and elastin; and
• fibroblasts.

Atherosclerosis

Smooth muscle cells can accumulate lipid and migrate into the subendothelial layer, which can then thicken and atherosclerosis can develop (Fig. 18g). This weakens the arterial wall, and can result in an aneurysm (swelling).

Atherosclerosis can lead to heart disease, stroke, and gangrene.

19 Capillaries, veins, and venules

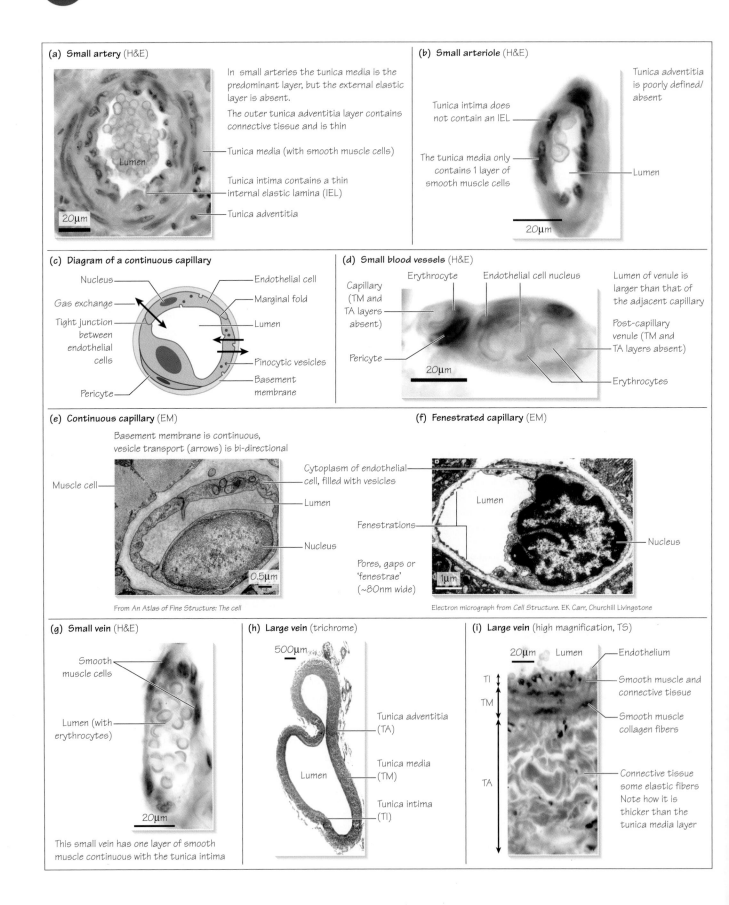

(a) Small artery (H&E)

In small arteries the tunica media is the predominant layer, but the external elastic layer is absent.

The outer tunica adventitia layer contains connective tissue and is thin

Tunica media (with smooth muscle cells)

Tunica intima contains a thin internal elastic lamina (IEL)

Tunica adventitia

Lumen

20μm

(b) Small arteriole (H&E)

Tunica adventitia is poorly defined/absent

Tunica intima does not contain an IEL

The tunica media only contains 1 layer of smooth muscle cells

Lumen

20μm

(c) Diagram of a continuous capillary

Nucleus

Gas exchange

Tight junction between endothelial cells

Pericyte

Endothelial cell

Marginal fold

Lumen

Pinocytic vesicles

Basement membrane

(d) Small blood vessels (H&E)

Erythrocyte

Endothelial cell nucleus

Lumen of venule is larger than that of the adjacent capillary

Capillary (TM and TA layers absent)

Pericyte

Post-capillary venule (TM and TA layers absent)

Erythrocytes

20μm

(e) Continuous capillary (EM)

Basement membrane is continuous, vesicle transport (arrows) is bi-directional

Muscle cell

Cytoplasm of endothelial cell, filled with vesicles

Lumen

Nucleus

0.5μm

From An Atlas of Fine Structure: The cell

(f) Fenestrated capillary (EM)

Lumen

Fenestrations

Pores, gaps or 'fenestrae' (~80nm wide)

Nucleus

1μm

Electron micrograph from Cell Structure. EK Carr, Churchill Livingstone

(g) Small vein (H&E)

Smooth muscle cells

Lumen (with erythrocytes)

20μm

This small vein has one layer of smooth muscle continuous with the tunica intima

(h) Large vein (trichrome)

500μm

Tunica adventitia (TA)

Tunica media (TM)

Tunica intima (TI)

Lumen

(i) Large vein (high magnification, TS)

20μm   Lumen

Endothelium

TI

TM

Smooth muscle and connective tissue

Smooth muscle collagen fibers

TA

Connective tissue some elastic fibers Note how it is thicker than the tunica media layer

Small arteries/arterioles

As arteries branch, and reduce in size, the outer elastic layer is lost, and the thickness of the tunica medica layer reduces in size.

Small arteries have the following characteristics.
- Diameter is about 0.1–2 mm.
- The smooth muscle layer (tunica media) is 5–10 cells thick (Fig. 19a).
- The tunica media contains mostly collagen, but some elastin.
- An internal elastic layer is present in the tunica intima.
- The tunica adventitia layer is thin, and contains connective tissue.

Arterioles have the following characteristics.
- Diameter is about 10–100 μm.
- The smooth muscle layer is 1–2 layers thick (Fig. 19b).
- An internal elastic layer is absent from the tunica intima.
- The tunica adventitia layer is thin and poorly defined.

In relation to their small diameter, the arterioles contain the greatest quantity of smooth muscle of any vessel.

This is important, because by contracting (vasoconstriction) and relaxing (vasodilation) their smooth muscle, these blood vessels control the blood supply into the capillary bed.

Constricting their lumens generates resistance to blood flow, and so these small arteries are known as 'resistance' blood vessels. They are the major determinants of blood pressure in the systemic circulation.

Capillaries

These are small, around 5–10 μm in diameter, just large enough to hold one red blood cell, although some specialized capillaries, such as those found in the liver, can be larger, 30–40 μm in diameter (see below).

The wall of the capillary contains flattened endothelial cells connected to each other by tight junctions (fascia occludens).

Capillaries do not have a tunica media or tunica adventitia layer (Fig. 19c–f).

The wall thickness of these vessels is only 0.5 μm, which facilitates gas diffusion across the capillary wall between the capillary and its surrounding tissue. Nutrients are exchanged by a mixture of gas exchange and pinocytosis ('cell drinking') in which the endothelial cells take up nutrients from the lumen via their apical surface, and secrete them into the surrounding tissue at their basal surfaces (or vice versa).

Types of capillary

There are three types of capillary: continuous, fenestrated, and discontinuous.

Continuous capillaries

In continuous capillaries (Fig. 19c–e, most common), tight junctions connect the endothelial cells to each other, and the underlying basement membrane is continuous. This type of capillary is found in muscle, the lung, and the central nervous system.

Continuous capillaries contain many vesicles, for transport of substances between the lumen and the surrounding tissue (Fig. 19e). They may also be surrounded by a pericyte, which contributes to new smooth muscle cells during development and in wound healing.

Fenestrated capillaries

Fenestrated capillaries are found in endocrine glands, the gut, and the gall bladder. They contain small pores (fenestrae) about 80 nm in diameter in the walls of the endothelial cells (Fig. 19f), which increases permeability between the capillary and the surrounding tissue. This allows exchange of macromolecules such as proteins (hormones) in addition to water and ions.

Discontinuous capillaries

Discontinuous capillaries also contain fenestrae but, in addition, the basement membrane of the endothelium is discontinuous. This type of capillary forms the liver sinusoids, found between liver hepatocytes. They contain particularly wide lumens (up to about 40 μm).

Sinusoids are also found in the spleen and bone marrow.

Capillaries drain into postcapillary venules and then into veins of increasing size. Arteriovenous shunts, direct connections between arteries and veins, can divert blood away from the capillary beds in some areas (e.g., the skin).

Veins

Veins are divided up into categories on the basis of size. These include small veins (postcapillary and muscular venules), and medium and large veins.

Postcapillary and muscular venules

These do not have a **tunica media** or **tunica adventitia** layer. They can be distinguished from capillaries because the lumen of these vessels is large compared to their thickness (Fig. 19d; compare the capillary and vein). Muscular venules are similar to postcapillary venules, but are surrounded by a thin layer of smooth muscle (1–2 layers, Fig. 19g).

Medium and large veins

Medium veins (diameter ~10 mm or less) mostly have names, and valves are common in these vessels, particularly in the lower limbs. Valves prevent the reversal of blood flow, due to gravity.

Large or muscular veins (diameter greater than 10 mm, Fig. 19h,i) are easily distinguished from arteries in sections by the following.
- The lumen of veins tends to be irregular, whereas that of arteries is regular.
- The tunica media is thinner compared to muscular arteries.
- The tunica adventitia is larger relative to the tunica media layer, and is the thickest layer. (Vasa vasorum can be present in this layer.)

The layer of smooth muscle in the tunica media layer is used to regulate the diameter of the veins. However, as blood pressure in the veins is lower, only a relatively thin layer is required.

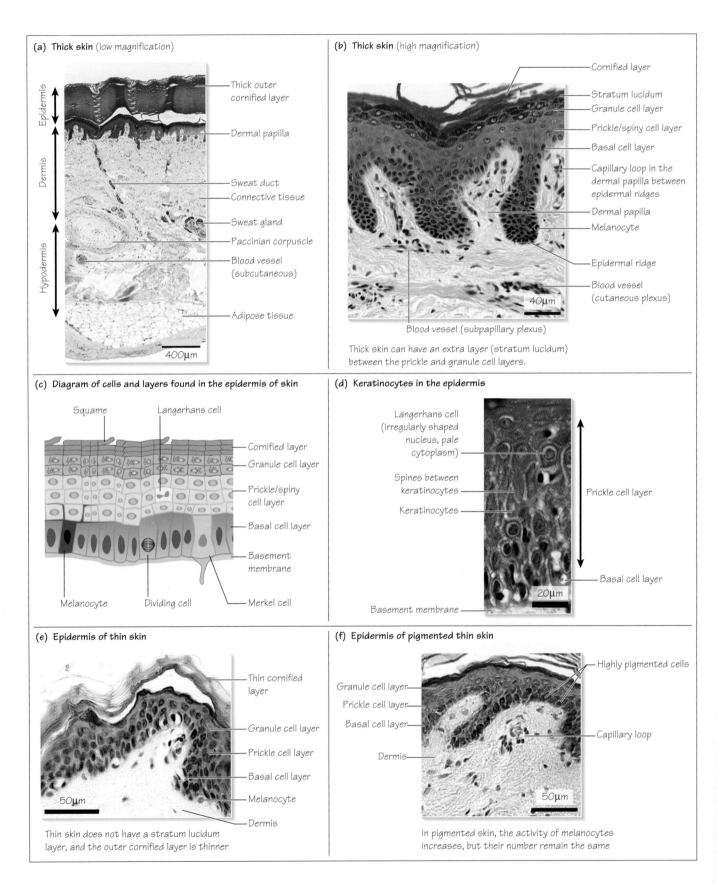

(a) Thick skin (low magnification)

Epidermis
Dermis
Hypodermis

Thick outer cornified layer

Dermal papilla

Sweat duct
Connective tissue

Sweat gland
Paccinian corpuscle

Blood vessel (subcutaneous)

Adipose tissue

400µm

(b) Thick skin (high magnification)

Cornified layer

Stratum lucidum
Granule cell layer
Prickle/spiny cell layer
Basal cell layer

Capillary loop in the dermal papilla between epidermal ridges

Dermal papilla
Melanocyte

Epidermal ridge

Blood vessel (cutaneous plexus)

40µm

Blood vessel (subpapillary plexus)

Thick skin can have an extra layer (stratum lucidum) between the prickle and granule cell layers.

(c) Diagram of cells and layers found in the epidermis of skin

Squame
Langerhans cell

Cornified layer
Granule cell layer

Prickle/spiny cell layer

Basal cell layer

Basement membrane

Merkel cell

Melanocyte
Dividing cell

(d) Keratinocytes in the epidermis

Langerhans cell (irregularly shaped nucleus, pale cytoplasm)

Spines between keratinocytes

Keratinocytes

Prickle cell layer

Basal cell layer

20µm

Basement membrane

(e) Epidermis of thin skin

Thin cornified layer

Granule cell layer

Prickle cell layer

Basal cell layer

Melanocyte

50µm

Dermis

Thin skin does not have a stratum lucidum layer, and the outer cornified layer is thinner

(f) Epidermis of pigmented thin skin

Highly pigmented cells

Granule cell layer
Prickle cell layer
Basal cell layer

Dermis

Capillary loop

50µm

In pigmented skin, the activity of melanocytes increases, but their number remain the same

The skin is the largest organ of the body (area ~1.6 m^2 in area, weight about 5 kg).

Functions of the skin

1 Protection: The thick epidermal layer, together with its waterproof coating, and pigment content, protect against ultraviolet (UV) light, mechanical, thermal and chemical stresses, and prevent dehydration and invasion by micro-organisms.

2 Sensation: Via receptors for touch, pressure, pain, and temperature.

3 Thermoregulation: Alterations in the peripheral circulation of blood regulate body temperature, as do sweat glands, hair, and adipose tissue.

4 Metabolic functions: Areas of the skin photosynthesize vitamin D, and lipids, including triglyceride (a neutral lipid).

All regions of skin contain the same three basic layers (Fig. 20a): an outer layer (the **epidermis**), an underlying **dermis**, and the innermost layer, the **hypodermis**.

The epidermis

This is the thin outer layer of the skin (Fig. 20b). It is a **stratified, squamous keratinizing** epithelium, which contains four layers of cells (sometimes five in areas of thick skin; Fig. 20c). It does **not** contain any blood vessels. The cells in the different layers change their appearance as they move upwards from the basal layer and differentiate.

Basal cell layer (stratum germinativum or stratum basale)

This consists of a single layer of cells, which lie closest layer to the underlying dermis. The cells adhere tightly to each other via desmosomes, and to the underlying basement membrane via focal adhesions (hemi-desmosomes). The basal cell layer contains several types of cell.

• **Stem cells:** which divide and renew the stem cell population and produce daughter cells (keratinocytes). They have a huge capacity for self-renewal: the outer layers of the skin turn over completely every 2 weeks.

• **Keratinocytes:** the most common cells in this layer (Fig. 20d). They divide 3–6 times before moving up into the prickle cell layer, and are cuboidal in shape with a pink cytoplasm and light purple nucleus.

• **Melanocytes:** pigment (melanin)-producing cells, derived from the neural crest in the embryo. There is 1 melanocyte for every 4–10 basal keratinocytes. Their numbers are similar from person to person, but their activity is much higher in dark skin (Fig. 20f). Melanocytes can be identified by their pale/clear cytoplasm and dark purple (basophilic) nucleus. Pigment is trafficked in vesicles (melanosomes) to the tips of long processes that penetrate into the prickle cell layer, and these are then engulfed (phagocytosed) by keratinocytes. The phagocytosed melanin then forms a layer in front of the nucleus, to protect against UV light.

• **Merkel cells:** rare neuroendocrine cells, which act as slowly adapting 'tactile' mechanoreceptors. They are most common in lips and the tongue, but are difficult to identify as they have a similar appearance to melanocytes.

In addition, there are free nerve endings (unmyelinated) which respond to pain and temperature.

Stratum spinosum (prickle cell layer)

This region consists of several layers of **keratinocytes**, and some **Langerhans cells**.

• **Keratinocytes** switch keratin expression from types 5 and 14 to types 1 and 10 as they differentiate. Keratin filaments inside the cell are connected to desmosomes to reinforce cell–cell junctions and make tight connections between the cells. These connections can sometimes be seen in histological sections as 'spines' in the light microscope, giving these cells their 'prickly' appearance.

• **Langerhans cells** are specialized antigen-presenting cells (dendritic cells), which account for 3–6% of the cells in the stratum spinosum layer (Fig. 20d). They contain long processes (dendrites) that ramify between the keratinocytes and contact other Langerhans cells to form a continuous network. When they are exposed to foreign bodies/antigen, they migrate out of the epithelium and into regional lymph nodes to initiate an immune response. Langerhans cells can be recognized by their round cell body, paler appearance of the cytoplasm, and oval-shaped nucleus.

Stratum granulosum (granule cell layer)

This layer lies on top of the stratum spinosum.

• It contains **keratinocytes** that have moved upwards and further differentiated into **granule cells**. They extrude specialized lipids in intracellular granules into the gaps between dead cells (squames) in the layer above. The proteins in these cells become cross-linked to form a tough proteinaceous scaffold. As they move upwards, these cells start to lose their nuclei and cytoplasmic organelles, and die. The dead cells become the keratinized 'squames' of the uppermost layer.

The stratum lucidum

This is a fifth layer occasionally found in thick skin between the stratum granulosum and the stratum corneum layer. It is thin and transparent layer and difficult to identify in routine histological sections.

The stratum corneum (keratinized cell layer)

This is the top, outermost layer and it consists of dead cells, that have become flatted and look like scales (or squames). These cells contain a tough layer of cross-linked keratins, on the inside bound to specialized lipids, on the outside to form a tough waterproof barrier. The squames eventually flake off (forming the main content of household dust).

The thickness of skin varies from 0.5 mm on the eyelids, to about 4.0 mm thick on the soles of the feet. Most of this difference is accounted for by the difference in thickness of the epithelium and, in particular, the cornified/keratinized cell layer (compare Figs 20a and 20e).

21 Dermis, hypodermis, and sweat glands

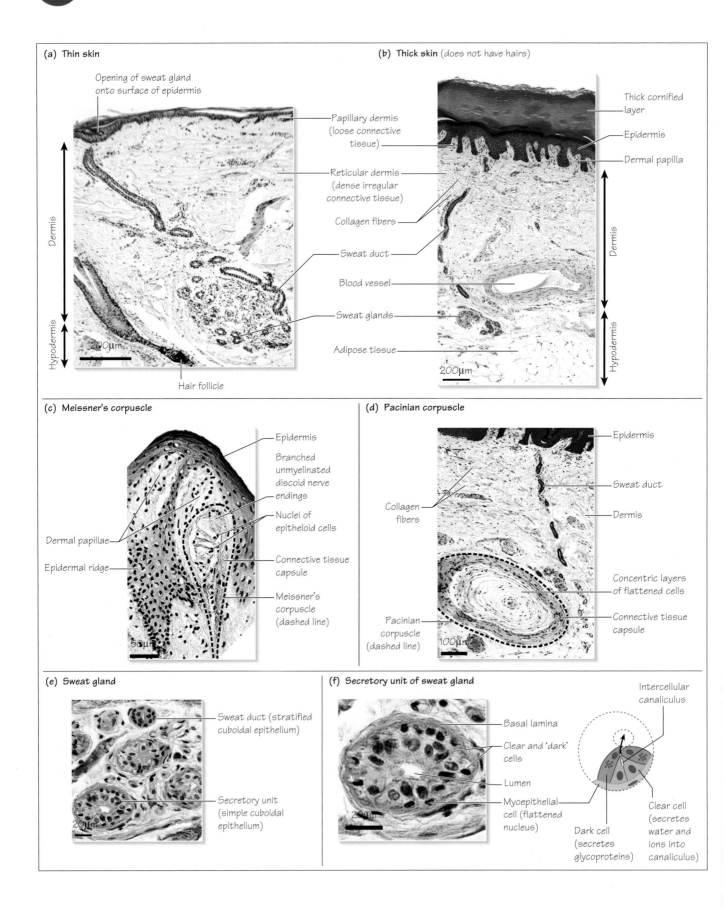

(a) Thin skin

Opening of sweat gland onto surface of epidermis

Papillary dermis (loose connective tissue)

Reticular dermis (dense irregular connective tissue)

Collagen fibers

Sweat duct

Dermis

Hypodermis

200μm

Hair follicle

(b) Thick skin (does not have hairs)

Thick cornified layer

Epidermis

Dermal papilla

Dermis

Blood vessel

Sweat glands

Adipose tissue

Hypodermis

200μm

(c) Meissner's corpuscle

Epidermis

Branched unmyelinated discoid nerve endings

Nuclei of epitheloid cells

Connective tissue capsule

Meissner's corpuscle (dashed line)

Dermal papillae

Epidermal ridge

50μm

(d) Pacinian corpuscle

Epidermis

Sweat duct

Dermis

Collagen fibers

Concentric layers of flattened cells

Connective tissue capsule

Pacinian corpuscle (dashed line)

100μm

(e) Sweat gland

Sweat duct (stratified cuboidal epithelium)

Secretory unit (simple cuboidal epithelium)

20μm

(f) Secretory unit of sweat gland

Intercellular canaliculus

Basal lamina

Clear and 'dark' cells

Lumen

Myoepithelial cell (flattened nucleus)

Dark cell (secretes glycoproteins)

Clear cell (secretes water and ions into canaliculus)

20μm

The dermis

This layer provides protection, sensation, and thermoregulation. It contains nerves, blood vessels, and fibroblasts that secrete the extracellular matrix, and fibers (collagen and elastin). It also contains sweat glands (at the border with the hypodermis), which open out onto the surface of the skin.

• The basal layer of the epidermis is folded into epidermal ridges, and between these ridges are folded regions of the underlying dermis, called dermal papillae.

• The dermal papillae are particularly prominent in thick skin (fingertips and the soles of feet).

The **dermal papillae**:

• increase adhesion between the dermal and epidermal layers;

• increase the overall surface area of the basal layer of the epidermis; and

• provide a large area of contact between the epidermis and blood vessels in the dermis.

The dermis is divided up into two main regions. The superficial region is called the **papillary dermis** and the deeper region is called the **reticular dermis** (Fig. 21a,b).

The **papillary dermis** is the region of dermis that is found in and close to the dermal papillae. This region accounts for about 20% of the dermis. It contains **loose connective tissue**, capillaries, and nerves, both of which extend up towards the epidermis between dermal papillae.

The **reticular dermis** is the remaining region of dermis excluding the papillary dermis. It contains a layer of **dense irregular connective tissue** that contains collagen fibers, woven into a dense network, and elastin. Both of these are secreted by the fibroblasts in this layer. These fibers give skin its strength and extensibility.

This layer also contains immune cells such as macrophages and fat cells (adipocytes), and the sweat glands, which are found deep in this region and in the hypodermis.

The hypodermis

This region of the skin mainly contains adipose tissue, and sweat glands (Fig. 21a,b). The adipose tissue is important for metabolic functions such as production of triglycerides and vitamin D.

The circulation of skin

• Arteries that supply the skin are found deep in the hypodermis (subcutaneous plexus).

• Branches from the arteries pass up towards the surface to form a deep (cutaneous) and a superficial (subpapillary) plexus.

• The pink color of skin is mainly due to the blood seen in venules.

• In cold conditions, blood flow to the superficial capillaries in skin is reduced to preserved core body temperature. In hot conditions, blood flow to the skin is increased and blood in superficial capillaries is cooled by the evaporation of sweat on the surface of the skin.

Encapsulated sense receptors in the dermis and hypodermis of skin

Meissner's corpuscles (Fig. 21c) are fast-adapting mechanoreceptors found in dermal papillae. They contain an unmyelinated nerve fiber (sensory neuron derived from the dorsal root ganglia) which branches repeatedly, forming disc-shaped nerve endings within a capsule of connective tissue. They are found in the fingertips, soles of feet, lips, tongue, and genital areas, and they detect shape and texture.

Pacinian corpuscles (Fig. 21d) are fast-adapting, pressure-sensitive receptors found in the hypodermis. The afferent nerve ending is encapsulated by multiple concentric layers of flattened cells, surrounded by an external capsule of connective tissue.

Ruffini's corpuscles are similar to Pacinian corpuscles, and are found in reticular dermis of skin and in joint capsules (not shown here). They respond to stretch, and adapt slowly to stimulation.

These three receptors, together with Merkel cells (see Chapter 20), are known as low threshold mechanoreceptors. Meissner's and Pacinian corpuscles both respond to initial skin contact.

The epidermis of the skin also contains non-encapsulated, or free nerve endings, which lack connective tissue and Schwann cells, and sense cold, heat, and fine touch.

Glands

There are two types of glands in the skin: **sweat glands** (Fig. 21e,f) and **sebaceous glands** (see Chapter 22). The cells that form these glands are derived from the epithelium.

Sweat glands are simple tubular exocrine glands that contain **secretory** and **excretory** portions.

• The **secretory** portion is found deep in the dermis/hypodermis.

• The **secretory** units have a simple cuboidal epithelium (Fig. 21e,f), which contains 'clear cells' that secrete (by exocytosis) water, Na^+ and Cl^-, and 'dark cells' that secrete glycoproteins to generate sweat. This type of secretion is known as merocrine secretion. Sweat can also contain urea, ammonia, and lactic acid, and it is hypotonic to blood plasma.

• Myoepithelial cells surround the secretory units (Fig. 21f). They contract to help the secretory units expel fluid.

• The **excretory** portion (ducts) lie throughout the dermis, and open out into coiled excretory ducts on the surface of the epithelium at sweat pores. A stratified (2 layers) cuboidal epithelium lines the ducts (Fig. 21e).

• Sweat evaporation is important for thermoregulation.

22 Hair, sebaceous glands, and nails

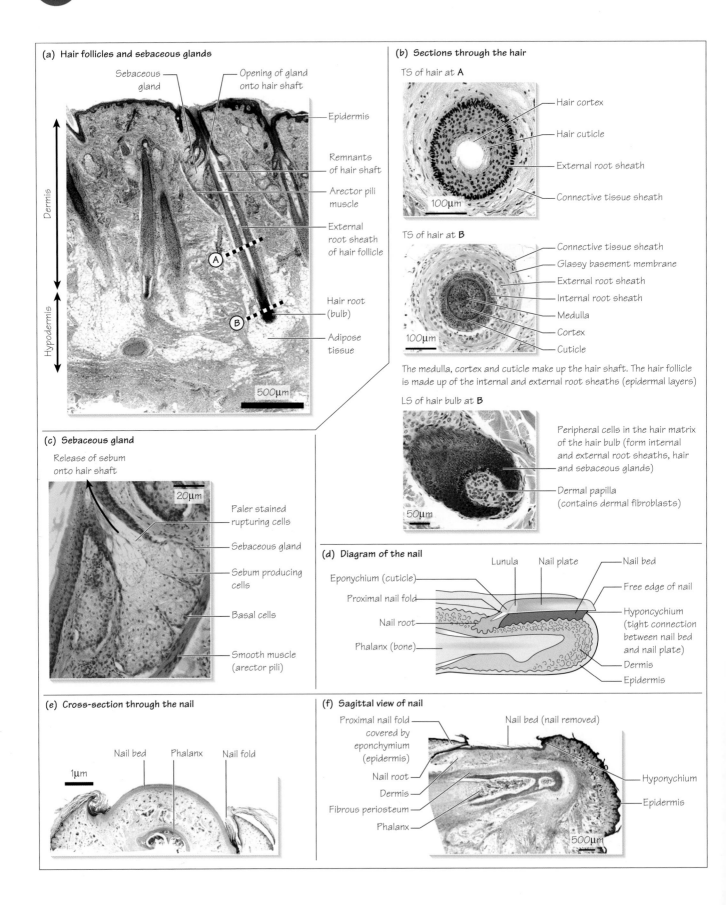

(a) Hair follicles and sebaceous glands

- Sebaceous gland
- Opening of gland onto hair shaft
- Epidermis
- Remnants of hair shaft
- Arector pili muscle
- External root sheath of hair follicle
- Hair root (bulb)
- Adipose tissue
- Dermis
- Hypodermis
- A
- B
- 500μm

(b) Sections through the hair

TS of hair at **A**
- Hair cortex
- Hair cuticle
- External root sheath
- Connective tissue sheath
- 100μm

TS of hair at **B**
- Connective tissue sheath
- Glassy basement membrane
- External root sheath
- Internal root sheath
- Medulla
- Cortex
- Cuticle
- 100μm

The medulla, cortex and cuticle make up the hair shaft. The hair follicle is made up of the internal and external root sheaths (epidermal layers)

LS of hair bulb at **B**
- Peripheral cells in the hair matrix of the hair bulb (form internal and external root sheaths, hair and sebaceous glands)
- Dermal papilla (contains dermal fibroblasts)
- 50μm

(c) Sebaceous gland

- Release of sebum onto hair shaft
- 20μm
- Paler stained rupturing cells
- Sebaceous gland
- Sebum producing cells
- Basal cells
- Smooth muscle (arector pili)

(d) Diagram of the nail

- Lunula
- Nail plate
- Nail bed
- Eponychium (cuticle)
- Proximal nail fold
- Nail root
- Phalanx (bone)
- Free edge of nail
- Hyponcychium (tight connection between nail bed and nail plate)
- Dermis
- Epidermis

(e) Cross-section through the nail

- 1μm
- Nail bed
- Phalanx
- Nail fold

(f) Sagittal view of nail

- Proximal nail fold covered by eponchymium (epidermis)
- Nail bed (nail removed)
- Nail root
- Dermis
- Fibrous periosteum
- Phalanx
- Hyponychium
- Epidermis
- 500μm

Hair

Hairs (Fig. 22a,b) are made up of **hair follicles** and **hair shafts**.

The **hair shaft** is made up of columns of dead keratinized cells (hard keratin) organized into three layers (Fig. 22b):
- a central **medulla**, or core (not seen in fine hairs);
- a keratinized **cortex**;
- a thin hard outer **cuticle**, which is highly keratinized.

Hair follicles are tubular invaginations of the epidermis, which develop as downgrowths of the epidermis into the dermis. The hair follicle contains the following.
- An **external root sheath** (**ERS**), which is continuous with the epidermis. This layer does not take part in hair formation. A **glassy basement membrane** separates the ERS from the surrounding connective tissue.
- An **internal root sheath** (**IRS**), which lies inside the ERS. The IRS contains keratinized cells derived from cells in the hair matrix. The type of keratin found here is softer than that found in the hair itself. The IRS degenerates at the point where the sebaceous gland opens onto the hair.

Hair follicle stem cells in the **hair matrix**, which is found in the **hair bulb**, are responsible for forming hair (Fig. 22b). The **stem cells** proliferate, move upwards, and gradually become keratinized to produce the hair. These stem cells also form the **ERS** and **IRS**, and sebaceous glands.

The dermis forms a **dermal papilla** at the base of the hair follicle/hair bulb, which provides the blood supply for the hair. It is separated from the hair matrix by a basement membrane.

Hair follicles can become inflamed, due to bacterial infections (e.g., *Staphylococcus aureus*), resulting in a tender red spot or pustule (folliculitus).

Contraction of the **arrector pili muscle**, a small bundle of smooth muscle cells associated with the hair follicle (Fig. 22a), raises the hair, and forms 'goose bumps'. This helps to release sebum from the gland into the duct, and to release heat.

Pigmentation of hair

Hair color depends on the pigment **melanin,** produced by melanocytes in the hair matrix. Differences in hair color depend on which additional forms of melanin, **pheomelanin** (red or yellow) and **eumelanin** (brown or black), are present.

The pigment is produced by melanocytes in the hair matrix, and is then transferred to keratinocytes, which retain this pigment as they differentiate and form hair.

In old age, melanocytes stop producing melanin, and hair turns white.

Hair growth

Hair follicles alternate between growing and resting phases.

Hair is only produced in the growing phase (this can be several years in the scalp).

Hair falls out in the resting phase. This can be permanent, resulting in baldness.

Cutting hair does not change its growth rate.

Sebaceous glands

These glands are branched, **acinar holocrine** glands found next to hair follicles (Fig. 22a,c).

The cells rupture to secrete an oily sebum into the lumen of the hair follicle (**holocrine** secretion).

The ruptured cells are continuously replaced by stem cells (**basal cells**), located at the edges of the gland.

Nails

Nails (or **nail plates**) consist of a strong plate of hard keratin, and they protect the distal end of each digit (Fig. 22d–f).

The **nail plate** is a specialized layer of **stratum corneum**. It is formed by the **nail bed** (**nail matrix**) underneath the nail plate. Proliferating cells in the basal layer of the nail bed move upwards continuously. As the cells move upwards they are displaced distally and gradually transformed into hard keratin, which lengthens and strengthens the nail plate. The tightly packed, hard, keratinized epidermal cells in the nail plate have lost their nuclei and organelles. Nails grow at a rate of about 0.1–0.2 mm per day.

The proximal end of the nail plate extends deep into the dermis to form the **nail root**. The nail root is covered by the **proximal nail fold**. The covering epithelium of this nail fold is called the **eponychium**. The outer thick corneal layer of the eponychium extends over the dorsal layer of the nail, to form the **cuticle**, which protects the base of the nail plate. If the cuticle is lost, the nail bed can become infected. The eponychium also contributes to the formation of the superficial layer of the nail plate.

The distal edge of the nail has a **free edge**. Here, the **nail plate** is firmly attached to the underlying epithelium, which is known as the **hyponychium** (*hypo* means 'below'). This region of epithelium contains a thickened layer of stratum corneum.

The tight connection between the nail plate and the underlying epithelium protects the nail bed from bacterial and fungal infections. If this connection is disrupted, then a fungal infection of the nail bed can cause **onychomycosis**.

Pigmentation of nails

The pink color of nails derives from the color of the underlying vascular dermis. The nail itself is thin, hard, and relatively transparent.

The white crescent at the proximal end of the nail is called the **lunula**. The underlying epithelium is thicker here, which explains the white color of the lunula. The increased epithelial thickness means that the pink color of the dermis does not show through.

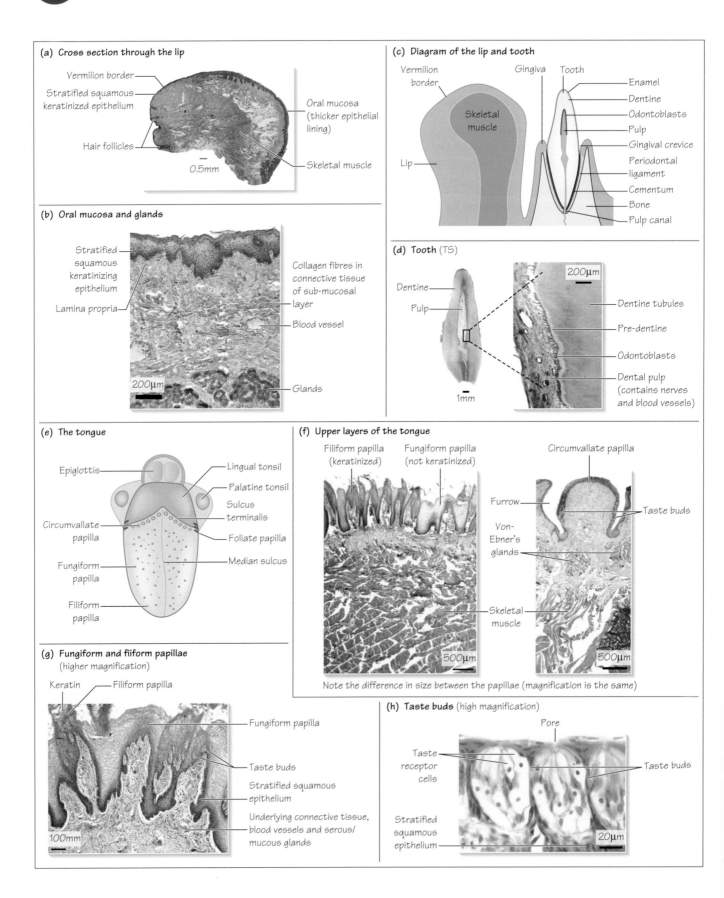

(a) Cross section through the lip

Vermilion border
Stratified squamous keratinized epithelium
Hair follicles
Oral mucosa (thicker epithelial lining)
Skeletal muscle
0.5mm

(b) Oral mucosa and glands

Stratified squamous keratinizing epithelium
Lamina propria
Collagen fibres in connective tissue of sub-mucosal layer
Blood vessel
Glands
200μm

(c) Diagram of the lip and tooth

Vermilion border
Gingiva
Tooth
Skeletal muscle
Lip
Enamel
Dentine
Odontoblasts
Pulp
Gingival crevice
Periodontal ligament
Cementum
Bone
Pulp canal

(d) Tooth (TS)

Dentine
Pulp
1mm
200μm
Dentine tubules
Pre-dentine
Odontoblasts
Dental pulp (contains nerves and blood vessels)

(e) The tongue

Epiglottis
Lingual tonsil
Palatine tonsil
Sulcus terminalis
Circumvallate papilla
Foliate papilla
Fungiform papilla
Median sulcus
Filiform papilla

(f) Upper layers of the tongue

Filiform papilla (keratinized)
Fungiform papilla (not keratinized)
Circumvallate papilla
Furrow
Von-Ebner's glands
Taste buds
Skeletal muscle
500μm
500μm

Note the difference in size between the papillae (magnification is the same)

(g) Fungiform and fiiform papillae (higher magnification)

Keratin
Filiform papilla
Fungiform papilla
Taste buds
Stratified squamous epithelium
Underlying connective tissue, blood vessels and serous/mucous glands
100mm

(h) Taste buds (high magnification)

Pore
Taste receptor cells
Taste buds
Stratified squamous epithelium
20μm

The mouth is the start of the digestive tract, a long muscular tube ending at the anus. A number of different glands are associated with the tract, which pour their secretions into the tube. In the mouth, these are the salivary glands (see Chapter 28).

The mouth performs a variety of tasks such as breaking up food, eating, speaking, and breathing.

The lip

The skin on the outer surface of the lip is a lightly keratinized, stratified squamous epithelium (Fig. 23a). The epithelial layer of the oral mucosa on the inside of the lip is thicker than that of the skin and is highly keratinized (Fig. 23a).

The 'free margin' of the lip is known as the **vermilion border**. This region looks red in a living person because it is highly vascularized.

The mouth

The mouth is lined by the oral mucosa (Fig. 23b), which consists of:
• a **thick stratified squamous epithelium**, which protects against the large amount of wear and tear that the mouth receives;
• an underlying layer of loose, vascularized connective tissue (**lamina propria**).

The epithelium is keratinized in less mobile areas (e.g., gums (gingivae), hard palate, and upper surface of the tongue) and not keratinized in more mobile areas (the soft palate, underside of the tongue, mucosal surfaces of the lips and cheeks, and the floor of the mouth).

The **submucosa** lies underneath the oral mucosa. This is a layer of dense irregular connective tissue, rich in collagen, containing salivary glands, larger blood vessels, nerves, and lymphatics. This layer is thin in regions overlying bone.

Teeth

Adults have 32 teeth, embedded in the bone of the maxilla (upper 16) and mandible (lower 16).

Teeth are divided into two main regions (Fig. 23c): the region below the gum contains one or more **roots**, and the region above the gum contains the **crown**.

Both the crown and the roots are made up of **three layers**.

Outer layer

The **outer layer** in the crown is a thin layer of **enamel**.

Enamel is a very hard, highly mineralized tissue, which is made up of crystals of calcium phosphate (99%). It does not have collagen as its main constituent, but does contain amelogenin and some enamelin.

Enamel is made by ameloblasts, tall columnar ectodermally derived cells, which are found on the outer surface of the tooth before the tooth erupts. After eruption, the ameloblasts die, which means that the enamel layer cannot be repaired.

The outer layer in the **root** is a thin layer of bone-like calcified tissue called cementum. Cementum is made by **cementocytes** (mesenchymally derived), and they become trapped inside the matrix of cementum.

Intermediate layer

In both the root and the crown, a layer of **dentine** is found underneath the outer layer of enamel/cementum. **Dentine** is calcified connective tissue that contains type I collagen (90%), and has a tubular structure.

• **Dentine** is made by odontoblasts, which lie between the central pulp layer and the dentine. Odontoblasts are derived from the cranial neural crest.
• Odontoblasts are columnar cells (Fig. 23d), and the apical surfaces of these cells is embedded in a non-mineralized pre-dentine layer. They secrete tropocollagen, which is converted to collagen once it has been secreted. The collagen fibers are then mineralized in the dentine layer.

Inner layer

Unlike bone, neither enamel nor dentine is vascularized. Therefore, the tooth has an **inner layer of pulp**, which contains the nerve and blood supply for the tooth, and in particular for the odontoblasts (once the tooth has erupted).

Gingival crevice: the basement membrane of the oral mucosa adheres to the surface of the tooth in the gingival crevice. A **periodontal ligament** connects the tooth to underlying bone. It has wide bundles of collagen fibers, and is embedded in a bony ridge (the **alveolar ridge**).

The tongue

The tongue (Fig. 23e,f) is a mass of striated muscle covered in oral mucosa. It is divided into an anterior two-thirds and a posterior one-third by a V-shaped line, the sulcus terminalis.

The mucosa covering the upper (dorsal) surface of the tongue is thrown into numerous projections called papillae (Fig. 23e,f). The epithelium of the oral mucosa is a stratified non-keratinizing squamous epithelium, and an underlying layer of lamina propria supports it.

There are three main types of papilla (Fig. 23f,g) on the dorsal surface of the tongue (a fourth type, foliate, is rare in humans).
• **Filiform papillae** (thread-like) are short whitish bristles. They are the commonest, appear white because they are keratinized, and contain very few taste buds.
• **Fungiform papillae** (mushroom-like) are small, globular, and appear red because they are not keratinized and are highly vascularized. They contain a few taste buds.
• **Circumvallate papillae** (wall-like) are the largest of the papillae. They are mostly found in a row just in front of the sulcus terminalis. Most of the **taste buds** are found in the circumvallate papillae in the walls of the clefts or furrows either side of the bud (Fig. 23h). **Taste receptor cells** in the taste buds only last about 10–14 days, and are continuously replaced by basal precursor cells. Serous (von Ebner) glands open into the cleft.

Tasting

Soluble chemicals (tastants) diffuse through the pore and interact with receptors on the microvilli of the taste receptor cells. This results in hyperpolarization or depolarization of the taste receptor cell, followed by transmission of a nerve impulse via the afferent nerve.

There are five types of tastes: sweet, sour, salty, bitter, and umami (monosodium glutamate). Some taste receptor cells respond to one of these and others to more than one.

Underneath the mucosa, most of the tongue contains longitudinal, transverse, and oblique layers of skeletal muscle (Fig. 23f). This organization of skeletal muscle gives the tongue its flexibility of movement. The tongue also contains connective tissue, which contains mucous and serous glands, and pockets of adipose tissue.

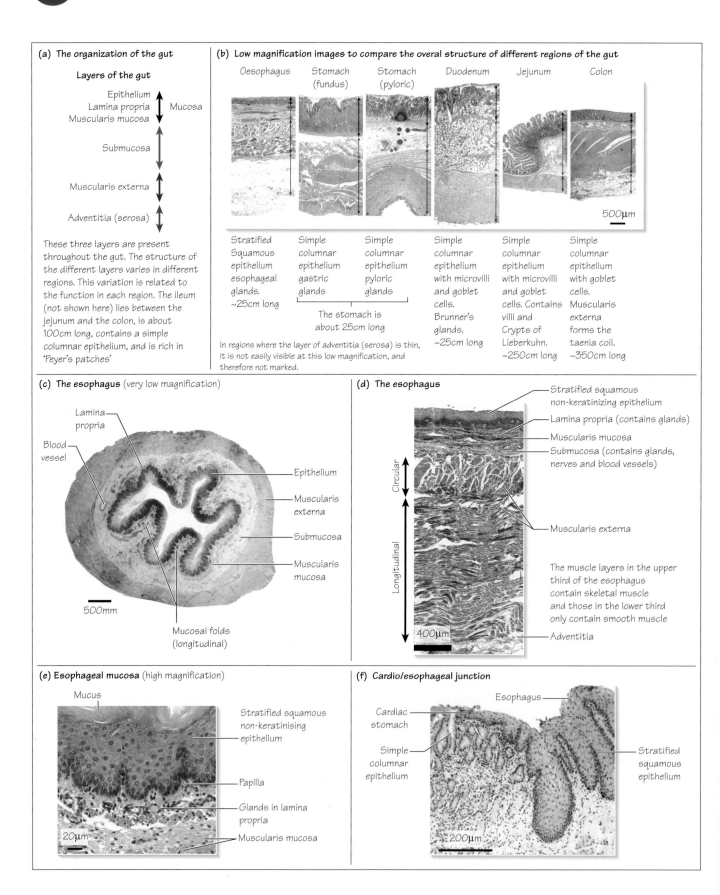

(a) The organization of the gut

Layers of the gut

Epithelium
Lamina propria ⟷ Mucosa
Muscularis mucosa

Submucosa

Muscularis externa

Adventitia (serosa)

These three layers are present throughout the gut. The structure of the different layers varies in different regions. This variation is related to the function in each region. The ileum (not shown here) lies between the jejunum and the colon, is about 100cm long, contains a simple columnar epithelium, and is rich in 'Peyer's patches'

(b) Low magnification images to compare the overal structure of different regions of the gut

Oesophagus	Stomach (fundus)	Stomach (pyloric)	Duodenum	Jejunum	Colon

500μm

| Stratified Squamous epithelium esophageal glands. ~25cm long | Simple columnar epithelium gastric glands | Simple columnar epithelium pyloric glands | Simple columnar epithelium with microvilli and goblet cells. Brunner's glands. ~25cm long | Simple columnar epithelium with microvilli and goblet cells. Contains villi and Crypts of Lieberkuhn. ~250cm long | Simple columnar epithelium with goblet cells. Muscularis externa forms the taenia coil. ~350cm long |

The stomach is about 25cm long

In regions where the layer of adventitia (serosa) is thin, it is not easily visible at this low magnification, and therefore not marked.

(c) The esophagus (very low magnification)

Lamina propria

Blood vessel

Epithelium

Muscularis externa

Submucosa

Muscularis mucosa

500mm

Mucosal folds (longitudinal)

(d) The esophagus

Stratified squamous non-keratinizing epithelium

Lamina propria (contains glands)

Muscularis mucosa

Submucosa (contains glands, nerves and blood vessels)

Circular

Longitudinal

Muscularis externa

The muscle layers in the upper third of the esophagus contain skeletal muscle and those in the lower third only contain smooth muscle

400μm

Adventitia

(e) Esophageal mucosa (high magnification)

Mucus

Stratified squamous non-keratinising epithelium

Papilla

Glands in lamina propria

Muscularis mucosa

20μm

(f) Cardio/esophageal junction

Esophagus

Cardiac stomach

Simple columnar epithelium

Stratified squamous epithelium

200μm

Organization of layers in the gut

The gut consists of four main regions, the esophagus, the stomach, and the small and large intestines.

Each of these regions consists of four main concentric layers (Fig. 24a).

Mucosa

The mucosa is made up as follows.

• **Epithelium:** The type of epithelium varies between different regions of the gut (Fig. 24b). The epithelium can invaginate into the lamina propria to form **mucosal glands**, and into the submucosa to form **submucosal glands**.
• **Lamina propria:** This is a supporting layer of loose connective tissue that contains the blood and nerve supply for the epithelium, as well as lymphatic aggregations.
• **Muscularis mucosae:** This is a thin layer of smooth muscle, which lies underneath the lamina propria, and contracts the epithelial layer.

Submucosa

The submucosa is a layer of supporting dense connective tissue, which contains the major blood vessels, lymphatics, and nerves.

Muscularis externa

This is the outer layer of smooth muscle. It contains two layers. In most regions of the gut, the smooth muscle fibers are arranged circularly in the inner layer, and their contraction reduces the size of the gut lumen. In the outer layer, the smooth muscle fibers are arranged longitudinally, and their contraction shortens the length of the gut tube.

Adventitia or serosa

This is the outermost layer, and contains connective tissue. In some regions of the gut, the adventitia is covered by a simple squamous epithelium (**mesothelium**), and in these regions, the outer layer is called the serosa.

The content and organization in these different layers varies throughout the gut (Fig. 24b), as each part of the gut is specialized for its particular role in processing food.

Nerve and blood supply to the gut

Arteries are organized into three networks:
• **subserosal** (between the muscularis externa layer, and the serosa/adventitia layer);
• **intramuscular** (through the muscularis externa layer);
• **submucosal** (in the submucosa).

Lymphatics are also present in the submucosa.

The gut is innervated by the autonomic nervous system (parasympathetic and sympathetic). Interneurons connect nerves between sensory and motor neurons in a submucosal plexus (Meissner's complex) and in the plexus of Auerbach (between the layers of circular and longitudinal muscle in the muscularis externa).

The esophagus

The esophagus is a muscular tube, about 25 cm long in adults, through which food is carried from the pharynx to the stomach.

The esophagus is highly folded (Fig. 24c), and can stretch out to accommodate food when it is swallowed and moved down to the stomach.

It has a protective type of epithelium (Fig. 24d,e), as it is open to the outside, and is exposed to a wide variety of food and drink (hot, cold, spicy, etc).

Swallowing is voluntary, and involves the skeletal muscles of the oropharynx. The food or drink is then moved rapidly into the stomach along the esophagus by peristalsis. A sphincter at the junction with the stomach (esophago-gastric junction) prevents reflux or regurgitation.

Mucosa

The **epithelium** of the esophagus is a protective **stratified squamous non-keratinizing** epithelium (Fig. 24d,e).

The basal layer contains dividing cells, which proliferate and move upwards, continuously replacing the lining of the epithelium.

Submucosa

The submucosa contains **loose connective tissue** that contains both collagen and elastin fibers. It is highly vascular, and contains esophageal glands, which secrete mucus into the lumen to help ease the passage of swallowed food, and the nerve supply for the muscle layers and glands. The esophageal (submucosal) glands are tubuloacinar glands, arranged in lobules, and drained by a single duct.

Muscularis externa

This muscular layer, lying underneath the submucosa (Fig. 24d), consists of an inner circular and an outer longitudinal layer of muscle.

In the top third of the esophagus, the muscle is striated; in the middle, there is a mixture of smooth and striated muscle; and in the bottom third, the muscle is entirely smooth.

The two layers allow contraction across and along the tube.

There is a sphincter at the top and bottom of the esophagus. The upper sphincter helps to initiate swallowing, and the lower to prevent reflux of stomach contents into the esophagus. Continuous chronic reflux (gastroesophageal reflux) causes Barrett's esophageal disease, in which columnar/cuboidal cells replace the squamous protective lining, possibly as part of a healing response. Goblet cells can also be present.

Adventitia

This layer contains connective tissue with blood vessels, nerves, and lymphatics.

Cardio-esophageal junction

As the esophagus enters the stomach, the epithelium changes from stratified squamous to simple columnar epithelium (Fig. 24f). The columnar epithelium is less resistant to acid reflux and can become ulcerated and inflamed, leading to difficulties in swallowing.

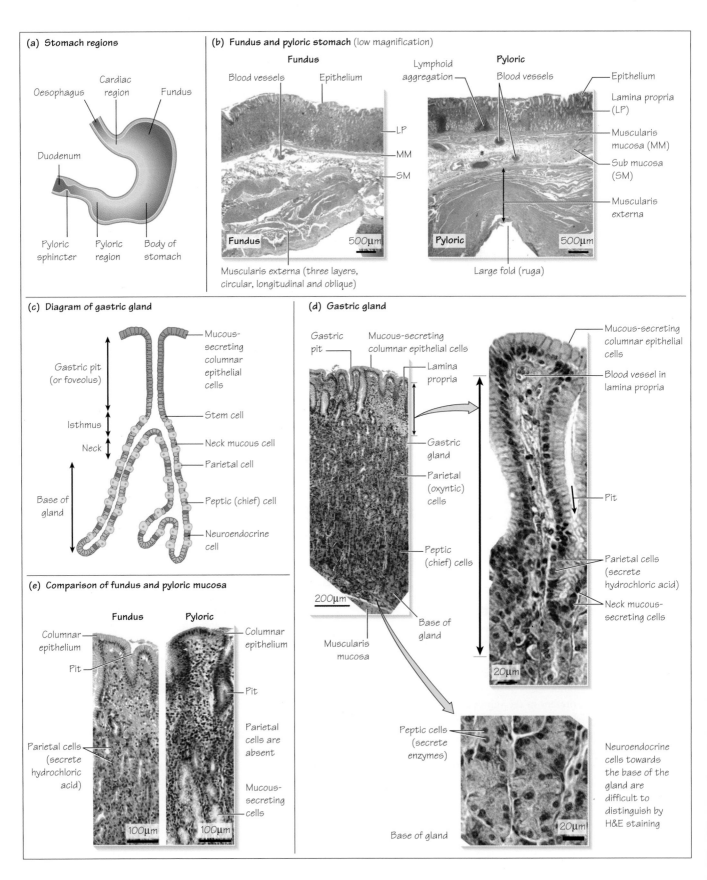

(a) Stomach regions

Oesophagus
Cardiac region
Fundus
Duodenum
Pyloric sphincter
Pyloric region
Body of stomach

(b) Fundus and pyloric stomach (low magnification)

Fundus
Blood vessels
Epithelium
LP
MM
SM
Fundus 500μm
Muscularis externa (three layers, circular, longitudinal and oblique)

Pyloric
Lymphoid aggregation
Blood vessels
Epithelium
Lamina propria (LP)
Muscularis mucosa (MM)
Sub mucosa (SM)
Muscularis externa
Pyloric 500μm
Large fold (ruga)

(c) Diagram of gastric gland

Gastric pit (or foveolus)
Isthmus
Neck
Base of gland
Mucous-secreting columnar epithelial cells
Stem cell
Neck mucous cell
Parietal cell
Peptic (chief) cell
Neuroendocrine cell

(d) Gastric gland

Gastric pit
Mucous-secreting columnar epithelial cells
Lamina propria
Gastric gland
Parietal (oxyntic) cells
Peptic (chief) cells
200μm
Muscularis mucosa
Base of gland

Mucous-secreting columnar epithelial cells
Blood vessel in lamina propria
Pit
Parietal cells (secrete hydrochloric acid)
Neck mucous-secreting cells
20μm

Peptic cells (secrete enzymes)
Base of gland
Neuroendocrine cells towards the base of the gland are difficult to distinguish by H&E staining
20μm

(e) Comparison of fundus and pyloric mucosa

Fundus
Pyloric
Columnar epithelium
Pit
Parietal cells (secrete hydrochloric acid)
100μm

Columnar epithelium
Pit
Parietal cells are absent
Mucous-secreting cells
100μm

The stomach is an expandable, muscular bag. Swallowed food is kept inside it for 2 hours or more by contraction of the muscular pyloric sphincter. It breaks down food chemically and mechanically to form a mixture called **chyme**. An empty stomach is highly folded (Fig. 25a). The folds (rugae) flatten out after eating so that the stomach can accommodate the food.

- **Chemical breakdown:** Gastric mucosal glands secrete **gastric juice**, which contains **hydrochloric acid**, **mucus**, and the **proteolytic enzymes pepsin** (which breaks down proteins) and **lipase** (which breaks down fats). The low pH of the stomach (~2.5) is required to activate the enzymes. The stomach absorbs water, alcohol, and some drugs.
- **Mechanical breakdown:** via the three muscle layers in the **muscularis externa**.

Anatomical regions of the stomach

- **Cardiac:** closest to the esophagus. It contains mucous-secreting cardiac glands.
- **Fundus:** the body or largest part of the stomach. It contains gastric (fundic) glands (Fig. 25b).
- **Pyloric:** closest to the duodenum, ending at the pyloric sphincter (Fig. 25b). It secretes two types of mucus and the hormone gastrin. The pyloric sphincter relaxes when chyme formation is complete, squirting chyme into the duodenum.

Body of stomach (fundus)

Mucosa

The **epithelium** of the fundus or body of the stomach is made up of a simple mucous columnar epithelium (Fig. 25d). The thick mucous secretion generated by these cells protects the gastric mucosa from being digested by the acid and enzymes in the lumen of the stomach. The epithelium is constantly being replaced, and cells only last about 4 days.

Tall columnar mucous-secreting cells line the epithelium on the surface of the stomach and the gastric pits. These cells secrete thick mucus.

Gastric glands

In the stomach, the epithelium invaginates to form **gastric glands** (Fig. 25c,d) that extend into the **lamina propria**. The glands open out into the base of the **gastric pits**. Cells lining the glands synthesize and secrete **gastric juice**. About 2–7 glands open out into a single pit. The stomach contains about 3.5 million gastric pits, and about 15 million gastric glands. The glands contain several different types of cells.

- **Tall columnar mucous-secreting cells** line the pit (Fig. 25d). Stem cells, neck mucous cells, and parietal cells are found in the neck and peptic and neuroendocrine cells are found towards the base of the gland (Fig. 25c,d).

- **Neck mucous cells** secrete mucus that is less viscid than that secreted by the **columnar cells** in the epithelium. Together, these mucous secretions help to protect the surface epithelium from being digested by the secretions of the gastric glands, by forming a thick (100 μm) mucous barrier. This barrier is rich in bicarbonate ions, which neutralizes the local environment. The bacterium *Helicobacter pylori* can survive in this mucous layer, and can contribute to ulcer formation and adenocarcinomas in the stomach.
- **Parietal (oxyntic) cells** secrete hydrochloric acid and are 'eosinophilic' (cytoplasm appears pink in H&E). Parietal cells also secrete a peptide that is required for absorption of vitamin B12 in the upper part of the intestine. Secretion is stimulated by acetylcholine and the hormone, gastrin.
- **Peptic (chief) cells** are found at the base of the glands. These secrete enzymes (pepsinogen, gastric lipase, rennin).
- **Stem cells** are found in the isthmus and not the base of the gland, as elsewhere in the digestive tract. Differentiating cells move up or down in the gland.
- **Neuroendocrine cells (G-cells)** are part of the diffuse neuroendocrine system, and secrete gastrin, which stimulates the secretion of acid by the parietal cells. These cells are found towards the base of the gland. They are 'basophilic' (the cytoplasm appears purple in H&E), and are difficult to distinguish from neck mucous cells in H&E.

The **muscularis mucosa** lies underneath the glands, and its contraction helps to expel the contents of the gastric glands. It has two layers, the inner is circular and the outer is longitudinal.

Submucosa

This layer contains blood vessels, nerves and connective tissue, but no glands.

Muscularis externa

In the stomach, this layer has **three** layers of muscle: an inner oblique layer, a central circular layer, and an external longitudinal layer. The contraction of these muscle layers help to break up the food mechanically.

Pyloric region of stomach

This region of the stomach is very similar to the body of the stomach (fundus). However, the mucosal layer is reduced in size, there are **no parietal cells**, and the glands are mostly full of mucous-secreting cells, which extend into the submucosa (Fig. 25e).

The muscularis externa layer in this region thickens to form the pyloric sphincter. This regulates the entry of chyme from the stomach into the duodenum, the first part of the small intestine.

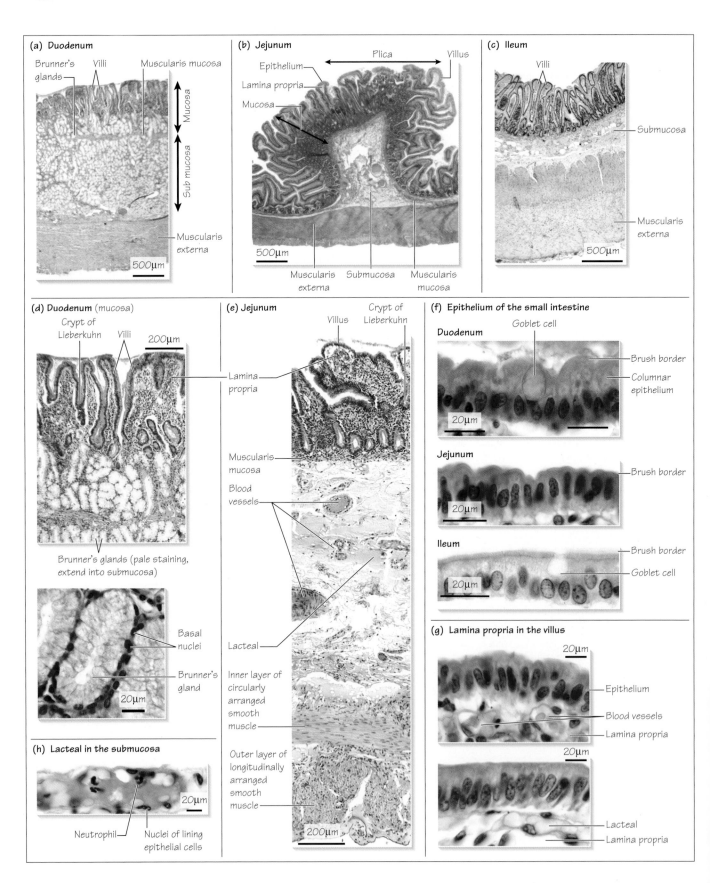

(a) Duodenum

Brunner's glands | Villi | Muscularis mucosa

Mucosa

Submucosa

Muscularis externa

500μm

(b) Jejunum

Plica | Villus

Epithelium

Lamina propria

Mucosa

500μm

Muscularis externa | Submucosa | Muscularis mucosa

(c) Ileum

Villi

Submucosa

Muscularis externa

500μm

(d) Duodenum (mucosa)

Crypt of Lieberkuhn | Villi | 200μm

Lamina propria

Brunner's glands (pale staining, extend into submucosa)

Basal nuclei

Brunner's gland

20μm

(h) Lacteal in the submucosa

20μm

Neutrophil | Nuclei of lining epithelial cells

(e) Jejunum

Villus | Crypt of Lieberkuhn

Lamina propria

Muscularis mucosa

Blood vessels

Lacteal

Inner layer of circularly arranged smooth muscle

Outer layer of longitudinally arranged smooth muscle

200μm

(f) Epithelium of the small intestine

Goblet cell

Duodenum

Brush border

Columnar epithelium

20μm

Jejunum

Brush border

20μm

Ileum

Brush border

Goblet cell

20μm

(g) Lamina propria in the villus

20μm

Epithelium

Blood vessels

Lamina propria

20μm

Lacteal

Lamina propria

The small intestine, 4–6 meters long in humans, consists of three regions.
- **Duodenum** (Fig. 26a,d) is found at the junction between the stomach and small intestine (25–30 cm).
- **Jejunum** (Fig. 26b,e) is the bulk of the small intestine (~250 cm long).
- **Ileum** (Fig. 26c) is found at the junction between the small and large intestine (~350 cm long).

The small intestine contains the same layers (**mucosa**, **submucosa**, **muscularis externa**, and **adventitia** or **serosa**) as the rest of the digestive tract.

Two features are important for digestion and absorption of food in the small intestine.

1 Enzyme and mucus secretion for digestion and to ease passage of food, and protect the lining of the intestine from digestion.

2 A large surface area for absorption, which is achieved by a series of folds.
  - **Plicae circulares** are large circular folds (Fig. 26b), which are most numerous in the upper part of the small intestine.
  - Folding of the mucosa into **villi** (Fig. 26a–c), small, finger-like mucosal projections, about 1 mm long (increase surface area by about ×10).
  - **Microvilli** are very small, fine projections on the apical surface of the lining columnar epithelial cells (Fig. 26e). This surface layer is commonly known as the 'brush border', and it is covered by a surface coat/glycocalyx.

Mucosa of the duodenum

The most obvious feature of the duodenum is the presence of **Brunner's glands**, which **are only found in this part of the small intestine** (Fig. 26a,d). These are tubuloacinar glands that penetrate the muscularis mucosa, reaching down into the mucosa.
- The pH of their mucous secretions is about 9, which neutralizes the acid chyme entering the duodenum from the stomach.
- The villi in the duodenum are shorter and broader than elsewhere in the small intestine, and have a leaf-like shape.
- The epithelium is made up of a simple columnar epithelium with microvilli and is rich in goblet cells, which secrete alkaline mucus that help to neutralize the chyme (Fig. 26f).
- Endocrine cells in the duodenum secrete cholecystokinin and secretin, which stimulate the pancreas to secrete digestive enzymes and pancreatic juice, and contraction of the gall bladder to release bile into the duodenum.
- The duodenum also receives bile and pancreatic secretions from the bile and pancreatic ducts.

Mucosa of the jejunum

The villi in the jejunum are long and thin.

The epithelium contains two types of cells (Fig. 26e,f): tall columnar absorptive cells (**enterocytes**) and **goblet cells**, which secrete mucus, for lubrication of the intestinal contents, and protection of the epithelium. Goblet cells are less common in the jejunum than in the duodenum and ileum. Intraepithelial lymphocytes (mostly T-cells) are also present.

The lamina propria in the core of the villus (Fig. 26g) is rich in lymphatic capillaries (lacteals), which absorb lipids, and in fenestrated capillaries.

Crypts of Lieberkuhn lie between the villi. These are simple tubular glands that contain the following.
- **Paneth cells:** defensive cells found at the base of the crypts. They secrete antimicrobial peptides (defensins), lysozyme and tumor necrosis factor α (pro-inflammatory). They stain dark pink with eosin in H&E.
- **Endocrine cells:** secrete the hormones secretin, somatostatin, enteroglucagon, and serotonin, and stain strongly with eosin.
- **Stem cells:** at the base of the crypts. They divide to replace all of the above cells, including enterocytes.

The **muscularis mucosa** layer at the base of the crypts contracts to aid absorption, secretion, and movement of the villi.

The pH of the mixture entering the jejunum is suitable for the digestive enzymes of the small intestine. Thus the jejunum is the major site for absorption of food, as follows.
- **Proteins** are denatured and chopped up by pepsin from gastric glands, and then further broken down by trypsin, chymotrypsin, elastase, and carboxypeptidases
- **Amino acids** are absorbed by active transport into the lining epithelial cells.
- **Carbohydrates** are hydrolysed by amylases, converted to monosaccharides, and absorbed by facilitated diffusion by the epithelium.
- **Lipids** are converted into a coarse emulsion in the stomach, into a fine emulsion in the duodenum by pancreatic lipases, and small lipid molecules are absorbed by the epithelium.

Other layers of the jejunum

The **submucosa** (Fig. 26b,e) contains blood vessels, connective tissue lymphatics (lacteals, lined by a simple squamous endothelium; Fig. 26f), and lymphoid aggregations.

Larger aggregations of lymphoid tissue called **Peyer's patches** are present (most common in the ileum).

The main blood supply for the small intestine enters via the submucosal layer in contrast to the stomach, where it enters via the serosal/advential layer.

The **muscularis externa** contains two layers of smooth muscle (Fig. 26b,e). The inner layer is circular, and the outer is longitudinal, and their contraction generates the continuous peristaltic activity of the small intestine.

The **outer layer of connective tissue** (adventitia) is covered by the visceral peritoneum, and is therefore called a **serosa**. It is lined by a mesothelium (simple squamous epithelium).

The ileum

This is the final region of the small intestine. It is similar to the jejunum, but has shorter villi, is richer in goblet cells and contains many more Peyer's patches (see Chapter 43).

27 Large intestine and appendix

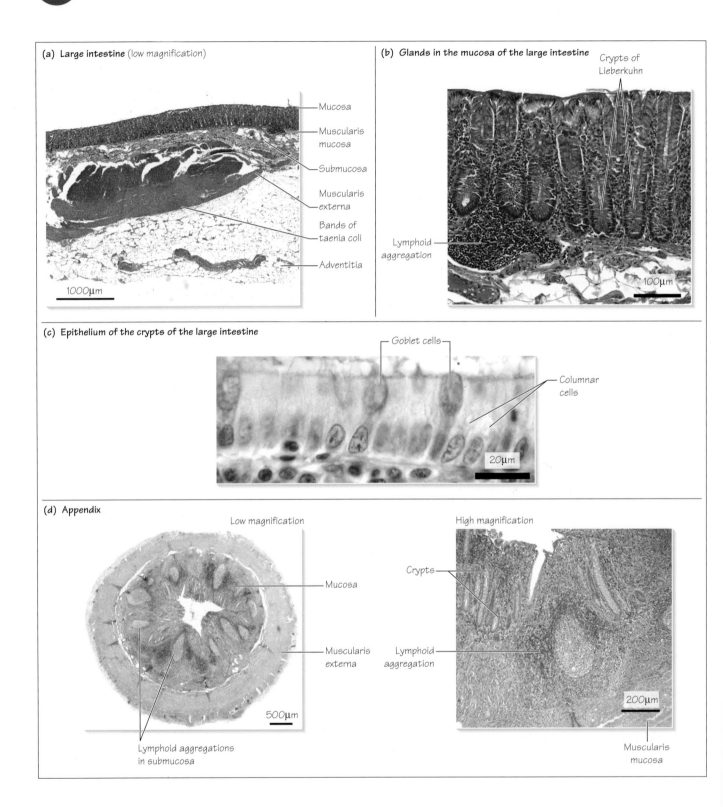

(a) Large intestine (low magnification)

- Mucosa
- Muscularis mucosa
- Submucosa
- Muscularis externa
- Bands of taenia coli
- Adventitia

1000μm

(b) Glands in the mucosa of the large intestine

Crypts of Lieberkuhn

Lymphoid aggregation

100μm

(c) Epithelium of the crypts of the large intestine

Goblet cells

Columnar cells

20μm

(d) Appendix

Low magnification

- Mucosa
- Muscularis externa

Lymphoid aggregations in submucosa

500μm

High magnification

- Crypts
- Lymphoid aggregation
- Muscularis mucosa

200μm

The large intestine

The large intestine consists of four areas: the cecum (including the appendix), colon, rectum, and anus.

Its main function is to absorb water, sodium, vitamins, and minerals from the luminal contents, which then become fecal residue. This highly absorptive feature is very useful for administering drugs (e.g., suppositories), when they cannot be taken orally. The large intestine does not contain any villi or or plica circulares.

The large intestine secretes large amounts of mucus, and some hormones, but no digestive enzymes.

Similar to the rest of the gut, the large intestine is organized into four layers (mucosa, submucosa, muscularis externa and adventitia; Fig. 27a).

Mucosa

The epithelium is folded to form tightly packed, straight tubular glands (crypts of Lieberkuhn; Fig. 27b).

The epithelium contains simple **columnar mucous absorptive cells** (Fig. 27c), which have short apical microvilli. These cells secrete a protective glycocalyx, which lines the epithelium, and absorb water, etc., (as outlined above). The epithelium also contains endocrine cells, basal stem cells, and numerous goblet cells. Paneth cells may be found in the cecum.

Goblet cells are found in the crypts and the columnar absorptive cells on the luminal surface.

The surface epithelial cells are sloughed into the lumen, and replaced every 6 days.

The mucosa also contains a **lamina propria** and a **muscularis mucosa**.

The lamina propria contains a thick layer (about 5 μm) of collagen, which lies between the basal lamina and the fenestrated venous capillaries. The thickness of this layer increases in hyperplastic colonic polyps. This collagen layer helps to regulate water and electrolyte transport between the epithelium and vascular compartments.

The core of the lamina propria does not contain any lymphatic vessels, but they are found in a network around the muscularis mucosa. This lack of lymphatics may help to explain why some colon cancers are slow to metastasize. The tumors have to enlarge in the epithelium and in the lamina propria, before they reach the deeper muscularis mucosa layer, where they can then gain access to the lymphatics.

Submucosa

The **lamina propria** and **submucosa** both contain aggregations of leucocytes (Fig. 27b) (gut-associated lymphoid tissue or GALT; see Chapter 43), but these do not form the dome-shaped structures of Peyer's patches (see Chapter 43).

The **submucosa** does not contain any glands.

Muscularis externa

The muscularis externa contains two layers of smooth muscle (inner circular and outer longitudinal). The outer longitudinal layer is arranged in three longitudinal bands that fuse together in a structure called the **taenia coli** (Fig. 27a).

At the anus, the circular muscle forms the internal **anal sphincter**.

Human appendix

The appendix is a blind pouch, which is found just after the ileocecal valve. It has the same layer structure as the rest of the digestive tract (Fig. 27d). However, the outer layer of muscle fibers in the **muscularis externa** is continuous.

Large amounts of **lymphoid tissue** in the **mucosa** and **submucosa** are arranged in follicles with pale germinal centers (Fig. 27d), similar to Peyer's patches (see Chapter 43). In adults, this structure is commonly lost, and the appendix is filled with scar tissue.

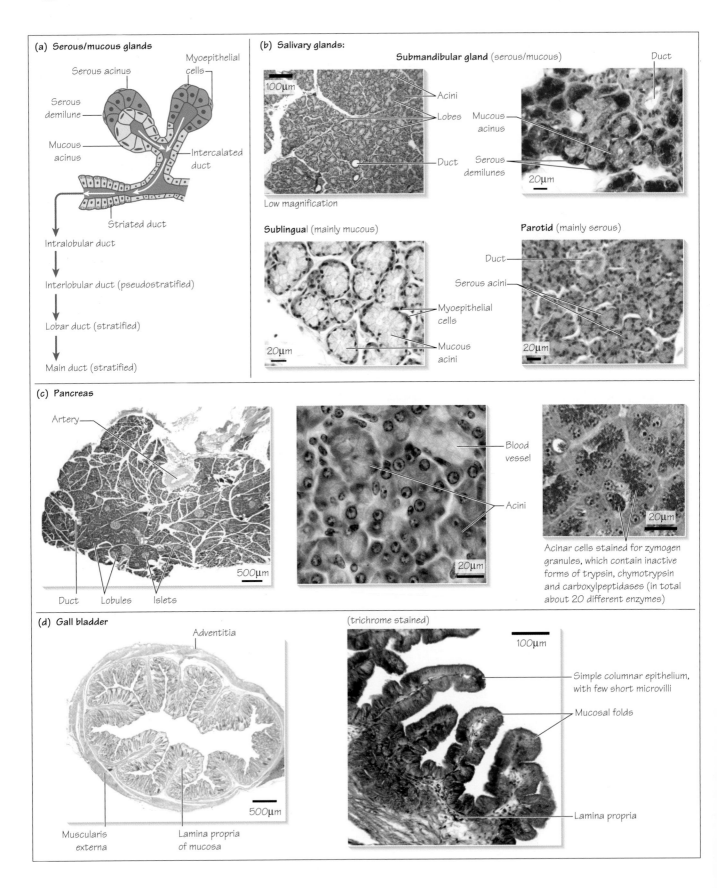

(a) Serous/mucous glands

Myoepithelial cells
Serous acinus
Serous demilune
Mucous acinus
Intercalated duct
Striated duct

Intralobular duct

↓

Interlobular duct (pseudostratified)

↓

Lobar duct (stratified)

↓

Main duct (stratified)

(b) Salivary glands:

Submandibular gland (serous/mucous)

Duct
Acini
Lobes
Mucous acinus
Duct
Serous demilunes

100μm
20μm

Low magnification

Sublingual (mainly mucous)

Myoepithelial cells
Mucous acini

20μm

Parotid (mainly serous)

Duct
Serous acini

20μm

(c) Pancreas

Artery
Blood vessel
Acini
Duct   Lobules   Islets

500μm
20μm
20μm

Acinar cells stained for zymogen granules, which contain inactive forms of trypsin, chymotrypsin and carboxylpeptidases (in total about 20 different enzymes)

(d) Gall bladder

Adventitia
(trichrome stained)

Simple columnar epithelium, with few short microvilli
Mucosal folds
Lamina propria

100μm

Muscularis externa   Lamina propria of mucosa

500μm

Salivary glands

There are three pairs of major **salivary glands: parotid, sublingual,** and **submandibular** (or **submaxillary**); as well as minor accessory glands in the mucosa, found in the oral mucosa. These glands secrete about half a liter of saliva per day.

Salivary glands are divided into lobules by connective tissue septa. Each lobule contains numerous secretory units or acini (acinus is a rounded secretory unit) and ducts (Fig. 28a,b).
• **Serous acini** secrete proteins in an isotonic watery fluid. **Parotid glands,** found on each side of the face, just in front of the ears, are mainly serous (which means that they stain strongly in H&E; Fig. 28b).
• **Mucous acini** secrete mucus, which contains mucin, a glycosylated protein that acts as a lubricant (note: mucus is the noun, and mucous is the adjective). **Sublingual glands,** found underneath the tongue in the floor of the mouth, are mainly mucous-producing (staining weakly in H&E; Fig. 28b).
• In **mixed serous-mucous acini,** the **serous** acinus forms a **demilune** around the **mucous** acinus, and its secretions reach the duct via canaliculi (small canals, which lie between the mucous cells). Myoepithelial cells around the acini contract to help with secretion. **Submandibular glands** underneath the floor of the mouth are mixed serous-mucous glands (Fig. 28b).
• The acini merge into **intercalated** ducts, which are lined by simple low cuboidal epithelium. Here the saliva is iso-osmotic with blood plasma (Fig. 28a).
• These empty into **striated ducts,** which resorb Na^+ and Cl^- ions (via active transport) to generate saliva, which is hypo-osmotic. Cells also secrete bicarbonate ions, and plasma cells in the ducts secrete IgA.
• The striated ducts lead into **interlobular** (excretory) ducts, which are lined with a tall columnar epithelium.
• In the mouth, the saliva forms a protective film on the teeth. Problems with the salivary glands can cause tooth decay and even yeast infections.

The pancreas

The pancreas is the main enzyme-producing accessory gland of the digestive system. It has both exocrine and endocrine functions. Endocrine functions are covered later (see Chapter 41). The pancreas consists of lobules (Fig. 28c), connective tissue septa, ducts, and islets of Langerhans (paler staining, endocrine regions of the pancreas, which makes up about 2% of the total).

Exocrine pancreas

The exocrine part of the pancreas has closely packed **serous acini,** similar to those of the digestive glands, and is thus a compound tubuloacinar gland (Fig. 28c).

The acini of the pancreas contain centroacinar cells. Their secretion (pancreatic juice) empties into ducts lined with a simple low cuboidal epithelium, and then into larger ducts with stratified cuboidal epithelium. This is then delivered to the duodenum via the pancreatic duct.
• Pancreatic juice is an **enzyme-rich alkaline fluid** (due to bicarbonate ions).
• The **alkaline pH** helps to neutralize the acid chyme from the stomach, as it enters the duodenum.
• The enzymes digest proteins, carbohydrates, lipids, and nucleic acids (including trypsin and chymotrypsin, which are secreted as inactive precursors, and activated by the action of enterokinase, an enzyme secreted by the duodenal mucosa).
• The release of enzymes is stimulated by cholecystokinin (CCK), which is secreted by the duodenum.
• The release of watery alkaline secretions is stimulated by secretin, which is secreted by neuroendocrine cells in the small intestine.

Gall bladder

The gall bladder is a simple muscular sac, attached to the liver. It receives dilute bile from the liver via the cystic duct, stores and concentrates bile, and delivers bile to the duodenum when stimulated (Fig. 28d).
• It is lined by a simple columnar epithelium (typical of absorptive cells) with numerous short, irregular microvilli (Fig. 28d).
• It is attached to the visceral layer of the liver, has an underlying lamina propria, but no muscularis mucosa or submucosa. The lamina propria contains many lymphocytes and plasma cells.
• The muscularis externa (muscle layer) contains bundles of smooth muscle cells, collagen, and elastic fibers.
• A thick layer of connective tissue, which contains large blood vessels, nerves, and a lymphatic network is found on the outside of the gall bladder. This layer is known as the adventitia, where it is attached to the liver.
• In the unattached region, there is an outer layer of mesothelium and loose connective tissue (the serosa).
• When fat enters the small intestine, enteroendocrine cells in the small intestine secrete the hormone CCK, which stimulates the contraction of the smooth muscle wall of the gall bladder. This expels the bile into the cystic duct, and from there into the common bile duct and duodenum. CCK production is stimulated when fat enters the proximal duodenum.
• The gall bladder can become inflamed (**cholecystitis**). A blockage of the cystic duct (**cholelithiasis**), due to gallstones, causes cholecystitis in most cases. Blood flow and lymphatic drainage from the gall bladder becomes compromised, causing tissue damage and death (necrosis). Gallstones usually consist of a mixture of cholesterol and calcium bilirubinate, which have become so concentrated that they precipitate out of solution.

29 Liver

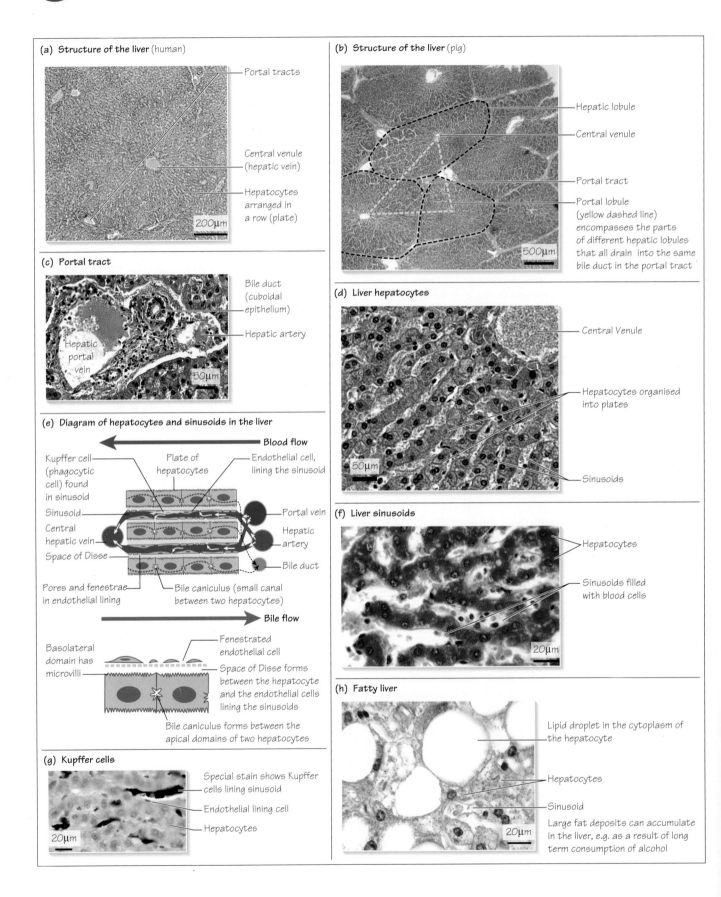

(a) Structure of the liver (human)

- Portal tracts
- Central venule (hepatic vein)
- Hepatocytes arranged in a row (plate)

200µm

(b) Structure of the liver (pig)

- Hepatic lobule
- Central venule
- Portal tract
- Portal lobule (yellow dashed line) encompasses the parts of different hepatic lobules that all drain into the same bile duct in the portal tract

500µm

(c) Portal tract

- Bile duct (cuboidal epithelium)
- Hepatic artery
- Hepatic portal vein

50µm

(d) Liver hepatocytes

- Central Venule
- Hepatocytes organised into plates
- Sinusoids

50µm

(e) Diagram of hepatocytes and sinusoids in the liver

Blood flow

- Kupffer cell (phagocytic cell) found in sinusoid
- Plate of hepatocytes
- Endothelial cell, lining the sinusoid
- Sinusoid
- Central hepatic vein
- Space of Disse
- Pores and fenestrae in endothelial lining
- Bile caniculus (small canal between two hepatocytes)
- Portal vein
- Hepatic artery
- Bile duct

Bile flow

- Basolateral domain has microvilli
- Fenestrated endothelial cell
- Space of Disse forms between the hepatocyte and the endothelial cells lining the sinusoids
- Bile caniculus forms between the apical domains of two hepatocytes

(f) Liver sinusoids

- Hepatocytes
- Sinusoids filled with blood cells

20µm

(g) Kupffer cells

- Special stain shows Kupffer cells lining sinusoid
- Endothelial lining cell
- Hepatocytes

20µm

(h) Fatty liver

- Lipid droplet in the cytoplasm of the hepatocyte
- Hepatocytes
- Sinusoid
- Large fat deposits can accumulate in the liver, e.g. as a result of long term consumption of alcohol

20µm

The liver is a major metabolic organ with numerous functions. It is involved in the following.

1 Red blood cell destruction and reclamation of their contents.
2 Bile synthesis and secretion.
3 The synthesis of plasma proteins (clotting factors and plasma lipoproteins) and secretion into the blood.
4 Glycogen storage and secretion of glucose.
5 The degradation of alcohol and drugs.

Structure of the liver

The liver is divided into hepatic lobules, each of which is surrounded by a thin layer of fine connective tissue. The hepatic lobules are not well defined by this connective tissue in most mammals (Fig. 29a), except in the pig, as shown here (Fig. 29b). A fine network of connective tissue fibers (type III collagen) provides support to the hepatocytes and sinusoid lining cells (not shown here). The lack of connective tissue makes the liver soft, and easy to tear in abdominal trauma.

Portal tracts at the **edges** of the lobules (Fig. 29c) contain terminal branches of the **hepatic artery**, the **hepatic portal vein**, and the **bile duct**.

The **hepatic vein** is found at the **center** of the lobule (Fig. 29d).

The liver is unusual because it has a **dual blood supply**. It receives:
• arterial blood from the **hepatic artery** (about 25% of the total blood flow); and
• venous blood from the **hepatic portal vein**, which contains nutrients absorbed from the gastrointestinal tract (about 75% of the total blood flow).

Blood leaves the liver in the **hepatic veins**.

Bile leaves the liver via hepatic ducts, merging into the **bile duct**. The bile is then delivered to the gall bladder for storage.

Importantly, **blood** flows from the portal tracts at the edges of the lobule **towards** the central vein.

Bile flows **in the opposite direction**, emptying into short **canals of Hering** close to the portal tracts, and then into the bile ductule in the portal tract itself.

Hepatic lobules

The hepatic lobules are made up of liver cells called **hepatocytes**, which are arranged in rows into 'plates' (Fig. 29d–f). The plates are one cell thick, and they can branch.

Blood from the hepatic artery and hepatic portal vein flows between the hepatocytes in **sinusoids**, which are a type of specialized capillary.

Endothelial cells that line the sinusoids are **fenestrated** and have a **discontinuous basement membrane**. These two features facilitate exchange between the blood and the hepatocytes.

The hepatocytes are separated from the lumen of the sinusoids by a thin gap called the **space of Disse** (Fig. 29e). Hepatocytes project microvilli from their basolateral domains into the space of Disse to increase the area for exchange of substances between the blood and hepatocytes.

Blood plasma filters through into the **space of Disse** between the hepatocytes and the sinusoids but blood cells or platelets do not. Thus hepatocytes are directly exposed to blood passing through the liver.

Phagocytic cells (**Kupffer cells**), which are derived from monocytes, also line the sinusoids (Fig. 29g). These cells remove worn-out blood vessels from the circulation.

Hepatic stellate cells (**cells of Ito**) are also found in the space of Disse. These store fat, and store and metabolize vitamin A.

Hepatocytes

Hepatocytes absorb substances from the blood, secrete plasma proteins (e.g., albumin, and some coagulation factors required for blood clotting), and make bile.

Hepatocytes are rich in **mitochondria**, **rough endoplasmic reticulum** (ER; for protein secretion) and **smooth endoplasmic reticulum** (for glycogen and lipid synthesis). Enzymes in the ER perform a variety of functions including synthesis of cholesterol and bile salts, breakdown of glycogen into glucose, conversion of free fatty acids to triglycerides, and detoxification of lipid-soluble drugs.

Hepatocytes are also rich in **peroxisomes** (for fatty acid metabolism). These vesicles perform a variety of oxidative functions, which results in the formation of a poisonous substance, hydrogen peroxide. This is then converted to water and oxygen.

Bile, synthesized by hepatocytes, is secreted into a system of tiny bile **canaliculi**. These do not have a duct-like structure but are formed by localized enlargements of the intercellular space between adjacent hepatocytes at their apical domains (Fig. 29e).

Bile is rich in water, bicarbonate ions (which make bile alkaline), cholesterol, bile salts, and phospholipids. It is important in emulsifying fats in the small intestine, for subsequent breakdown by enzymes (lipases) into fatty acids and monoglycerides. It also contains conjugated bilirubin, a byproduct of the breakdown of red blood cells, for excretion.

One important function of hepatocytes is to metabolize alcohol. Ethanol, taken up by the cells, is oxidized to acetaldehyde by alcohol dehydrogenase in the cytoplasm, and then converted to acetate in mitochondria and in peroxisomes. Excess acetate damages mitochondria, and excess hydrogen peroxide damages the hepatocyte membranes.

Long-term alcohol use results in a fatty liver (Fig. 29h), and can lead to cirrhosis (proliferation of the collagen fiber network) or even carcinoma. The increase in collagen fibers results from the transformation of the **cells of Ito**, which contribute to formation of scar tissue (fibrosis) in the liver.

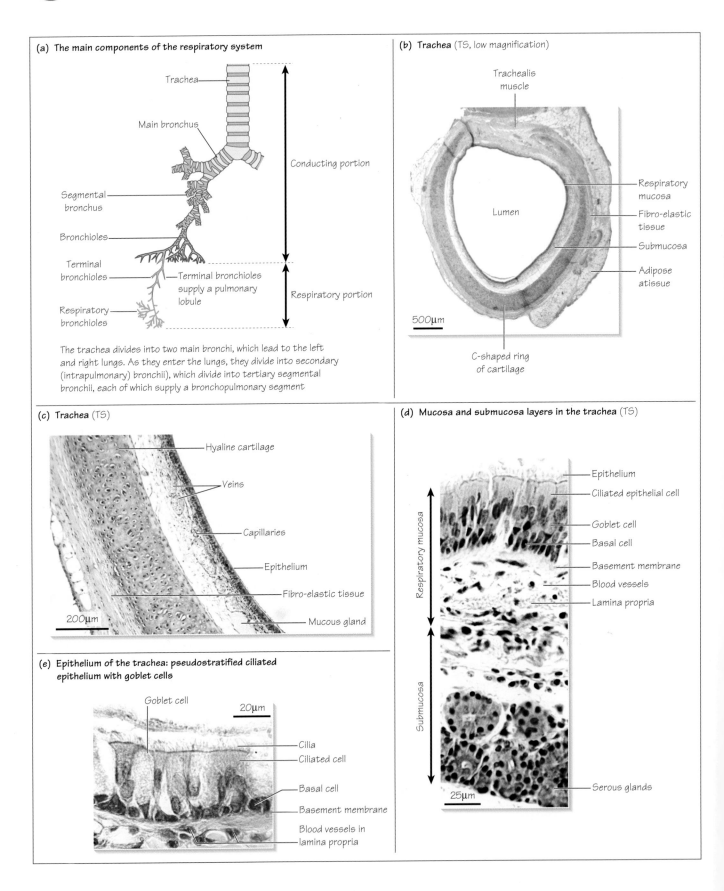

(a) The main components of the respiratory system

Trachea

Main bronchus

Segmental bronchus

Bronchioles

Terminal bronchioles

Respiratory bronchioles

Terminal bronchioles supply a pulmonary lobule

Conducting portion

Respiratory portion

The trachea divides into two main bronchi, which lead to the left and right lungs. As they enter the lungs, they divide into secondary (intrapulmonary) bronchii), which divide into tertiary segmental bronchii, each of which supply a bronchopulmonary segment

(b) Trachea (TS, low magnification)

Trachealis muscle

Lumen

Respiratory mucosa

Fibro-elastic tissue

Submucosa

Adipose atissue

C-shaped ring of cartilage

500μm

(c) Trachea (TS)

Hyaline cartilage

Veins

Capillaries

Epithelium

Fibro-elastic tissue

Mucous gland

200μm

(d) Mucosa and submucosa layers in the trachea (TS)

Respiratory mucosa

Submucosa

Epithelium

Ciliated epithelial cell

Goblet cell

Basal cell

Basement membrane

Blood vessels

Lamina propria

Serous glands

25μm

(e) Epithelium of the trachea: pseudostratified ciliated epithelium with goblet cells

Goblet cell

20μm

Cilia

Ciliated cell

Basal cell

Basement membrane

Blood vessels in lamina propria

The respiratory system consists of two major components, the conducting portion and the respiratory portion (Fig. 35a). The conducting portion includes the nasal cavities, nasopharynx, larynx, trachea, and bronchi.

Conducting portion

The conducting portion **transports** the inhaled and the exhaled gases between atmosphere and the respiratory portion.

The conducting portion conditions the inhaled air before it reaches the respiratory portion in the following way.
- **Filtering:** Viscid mucus secreted into the lumen traps foreign particulate matter, and the cilia on epithelium move the mucus upwards, away from the respiratory portion. The mucus is eventually swallowed.
- **Humidifying:** Secretions of watery mucus into the lumen humidify the inhaled air.
- **Warming:** A rich blood supply underneath the epithelium warms the air.

The conducting portion consists of the upper respiratory tract: the nasal cavities, nasopharynx, mouth, larynx, trachea, bronchii, and bronchioles (Fig. 30a).

Basic structure of the conducting portion

- **Mucosa:** lining epithelium and underlying layer of connective tissue (lamina propria).
- **Submucosa:** layer of connective tissue that contains glands and blood vessels lying underneath the respiratory mucosa.
- **Cartilage and/or muscle:** lies underneath the submucosa.
- **Adventitia:** the external layer of connective tissue.

Nasal cavities, nasopharynx, and larynx

The nasal cavities are lined by a ciliated epithelium. They contain olfactory receptors, which are bipolar neurons, with a non-motile cilium on their surface. These receptors detect smells or odors, bound to proteins in the fluid on the surface of the epithelium. Signals are sent down the bipolar neurons for processing in the olfactory bulb.

The trachea

The trachea is a wide (~2cm) flexible tube about 10cm long (Fig. 34b). The lumen of the tube is kept open by up to 20 rings of **hyaline cartilage**, which are organized into **C-shaped rings**. It forms the major part of the conduction portion of the respiratory system.

The gaps between the C-shaped rings are filled with **fibroelastic tissue** and the **trachealis** muscle (a bundle of smooth muscle). This arrangement holds the airway open, and in addition allows flexibility during inspiration and expiration.

Respiratory mucosa

The lumen is lined by **respiratory mucosa**, which is made up of the epithelium and underlying lamina propria (Fig. 30c,d).

The **epithelium** consists of basal cells, ciliated columnar cells, and interspersed goblet cells (Fig. 30e). Basal cells (about 30%) do not extend all the way up from the basal lamina to the lumen. These cells act as 'stem' cells for the epithelium. Ciliated cells (30%) extend from the basal lamina to the lumen, as do goblet cells.

The nuclei of the basal cells, columnar cells, and the goblet cells are at different levels, giving this epithelium the appearance of being stratified, but it is a single layer of cells. Hence it is a **pseudostratified ciliated epithelium with goblet cells** (see Chapter 7).

The nuclei of the goblet cells stain darkly and have a characteristic cup-like shape. Those of the ciliated cells are paler, and centrally localized.

The underlying basement membrane is thick.

The **lamina propria** is a layer of loose connective tissue underneath the epithelium, which is highly vascularized, to warm the inhaled air.

Submucosa

The **submucosa** contains seromucous glands, which secrete mucus onto the lining of the trachea. These secretions, in addition to the mucus secreted by goblet cells, provide a thick protective layer over the epithelium. The serous glands (which stain strongly in H&E) secrete a watery secretion. The mucous glands (which stain weakly in H&E) secrete a viscid mucous secretion.

Cartilage

The layer of cartilage is surrounded by fibro-elastic tissue in the adventitia, which merges with the lung tissue (parenchyma).

31 Bronchi, bronchioles, and the respiratory portion of the lungs

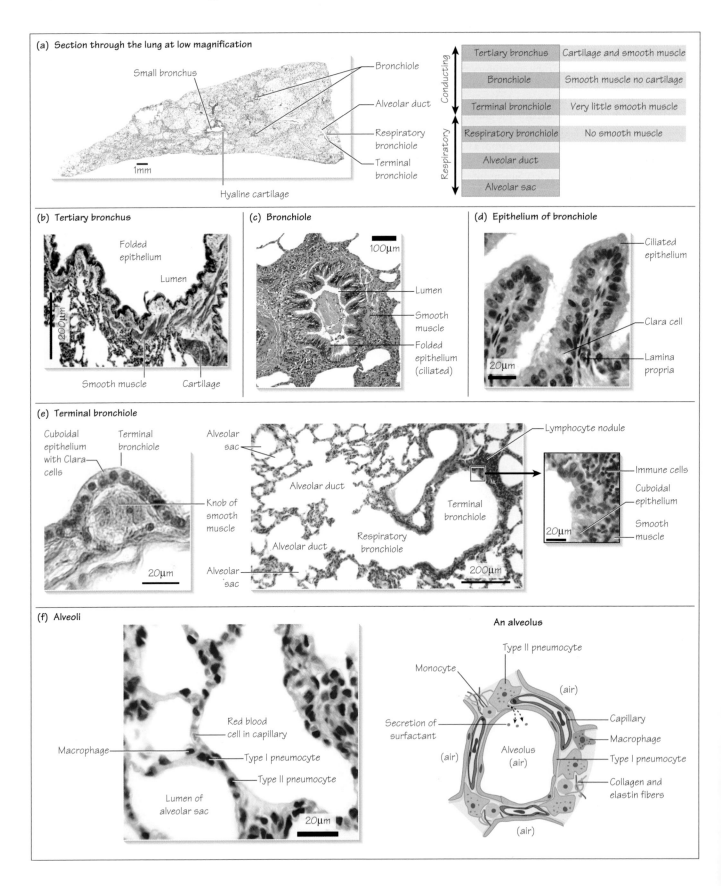

(a) Section through the lung at low magnification

Small bronchus
Bronchiole
Alveolar duct
Respiratory bronchiole
Terminal bronchiole
Hyaline cartilage
1mm

Conducting	Tertiary bronchus	Cartilage and smooth muscle
	Bronchiole	Smooth muscle no cartilage
	Terminal bronchiole	Very little smooth muscle
Respiratory	Respiratory bronchiole	No smooth muscle
	Alveolar duct	
	Alveolar sac	

(b) Tertiary bronchus

Folded epithelium
Lumen
200μm
Smooth muscle
Cartilage

(c) Bronchiole

100μm
Lumen
Smooth muscle
Folded epithelium (ciliated)

(d) Epithelium of bronchiole

Ciliated epithelium
Clara cell
Lamina propria
20μm

(e) Terminal bronchiole

Cuboidal epithelium with Clara cells
Terminal bronchiole
Knob of smooth muscle
20μm

Alveolar sac
Alveolar duct
Respiratory bronchiole
Alveolar sac
Terminal bronchiole
200μm

Lymphocyte nodule
Immune cells
Cuboidal epithelium
Smooth muscle
20μm

(f) Alveoli

Macrophage
Red blood cell in capillary
Type I pneumocyte
Type II pneumocyte
Lumen of alveolar sac
20μm

An alveolus

Monocyte
Type II pneumocyte
(air)
Secretion of surfactant
Capillary
Macrophage
Type I pneumocyte
Alveolus (air)
(air)
Collagen and elastin fibers
(air)

 Histology at a Glance, 1st edition. © Michelle Peckham. Published 2011 by Blackwell Publishing Ltd.

The trachea branches into two main bronchi, then into segmental bronchi, in which the diameter gradually reduces in size, and ends in tertiary bronchi. These then divide into bronchioles, ending at terminal bronchioles, which are the final part of the conducting system.

Terminal bronchioles lead into respiratory bronchioles, which form the start of the respiratory portion, which branch into alveolar ducts, alveoli sacs, and alveoli (Fig. 31a).

All of these structures are lined by a ciliated epithelium, but the number of goblet and other secretory cells is gradually reduced, as is the amount of cartilage. Bronchioles, and alveolar ducts and sacs, do not contain any cartilage.

The different structures can be distinguished from each other from their diameter, organization of the respiratory mucosa, submucosa and the presence/absence of cartilage and/or smooth muscle layers.

Tertiary bronchi

- All of the bronchi contain cartilage, and they contain glands in the submucosa.
- Tertiary bronchi are the smallest type of bronchus and the diameter of their lumen is about 1 mm.
- The epithelium of the mucosa is ciliated and there are only a few goblet cells.
- The epithelium is classified as a ciliated tall columnar epithelium.
- The underlying lamina propria is thin and sero-mucous glands are sparse.
- The mucosa is usually folded.
- The framework of cartilage is reduced to a few small fragments (Fig. 31b), and there is a layer of smooth muscle that encircles the bronchi.
- Contraction of the smooth muscle controls the diameter of the airway.

Bronchioles

- The diameter of bronchioles is less than 1 mm.
- Bronchioles do not contain any cartilage. A ring of smooth muscle surrounds the bronchioles, and contraction of this muscle regulates their diameter (Fig. 31c).
- Contraction is controlled by the vagus nerve (parasympathetic).
- The epithelium is ciliated and columnar, or cuboidal and there is a thin underlying lamina propria (Fig. 31d).
- **Clara cells** may be present, instead of goblet cells. These are non-ciliated cells, which secrete a protein, glycoprotein, and lipid-rich secretion into the airways, which may act as a surfactant. They also secrete the detoxifying compound cytochrome p450, and may help to regenerate the epithelium of small airways, when damaged.
- A network of elastic fibers attaches the bronchioles to the surrounding lung tissue. This keeps their lumens open, in the absence of cartilage.
- **Terminal bronchioles** are the smallest type of bronchiole. They are very small in diameter, contain a cuboidal epithelium with some Clara cells, and smooth muscle is much reduced. These structures lead to respiratory bronchioles that connect with the respiratory portion of the lungs.

Respiratory portion

The respiratory portion contains respiratory bronchioles, alveolar ducts, alveolar sacs, and alveoli. Alveoli contain the main interface for **passive exchange** of gases between atmosphere and blood. It consists of an epithelium and an underlying lamina propria, but no muscle or cartilage.

Respiratory bronchioles

Respiratory bronchioles only contain a layer of mucosa (epithelium and underlying lamina propria).

Single alveoli branch off their walls.

Respiratory bronchioles have a ciliated cuboidal epithelium, which also contains some secretory cells (**Clara** cells).

The respiratory bronchioles lead into alveolar ducts (which are surrounded by smooth muscle, elastin, and collagen), and these lead into the alveolar sacs.

Alveoli sacs and alveoli

The alveolar sacs contain several alveoli, surrounded by blood vessels, which are derived from the pulmonary artery.

The barrier between the lumen of the alveolar sac and the lumen of the capillary (the alveolar-capillary barrier) is very thin, varying from 0.2 to 2.5 μm.

This narrow barrier allows the rapid transport of gases (carbon dioxide and oxygen) from the air in the lumen of the alveoli into the blood capillaries and vice versa.

The alveoli contain two main types of cells, type I and type II pneumocytes.

Type I pneumocytes

These are large flattened cells, which make up 95% of the total alveolar area.

Tight junctions connect these cells to each other.

Their cell walls are fused to those of the capillary endothelial cells with only a very thin basement membrane between them.

This arrangement generates the very thin gap across which oxygen and carbon dioxide can rapidly diffuse.

Type II pneumocytes

These cells make up 60% of the total number of cells, but only 5% of the total alveolar area.

They secrete 'surfactant'. This stops the thin alveolar walls from sticking together during inspiration and expiration, by overcoming the effects of surface tension.

90% of surfactant consists of phospholipids, and 10% of proteins, including apoliproteins.

These are released by exocytosis onto the alveolar surface to form a tubular lattice of lipoprotein.

These cells are connected to other cells in the epithelium by tight junctions.

Macrophages/monocytes

Macrophages ('dust cells'), derived from monocytes, migrate into the lumen of the alveoli.

They act as efficient scavengers, by mounting an immediate response to any bacteria or foreign bodies that reaches the alveoli. They are very common but are gradually lost, as the cells move upwards towards the pharynx.

Special stains are needed to unambiguously identify the different cells.

32

Renal corpuscle

(a) The functional unit of the kidney: nephron and collecting tubule

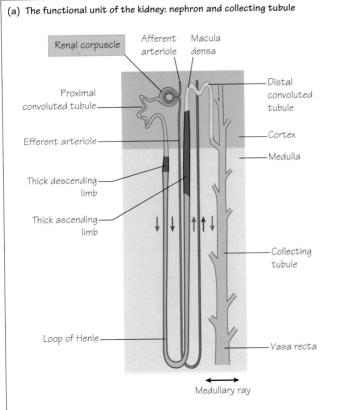

Renal corpuscle

Afferent arteriole

Macula densa

Proximal convoluted tubule

Efferent arteriole

Thick descending limb

Thick ascending limb

Loop of Henle

Distal convoluted tubule

Cortex

Medulla

Collecting tubule

Vasa recta

Medullary ray

There are two types of nephron. The one shown in the diagram is a juxtamedullary nephron, where the corpuscle is close to the medulla, and the loop of Henle enters deep into the medulla. The arteriole that supplies this corpuscle forms the 'vasa recta', capillary loops that enter the medulla and form a network around the collecting ducts and loop of Henle. There are also cortical nephrons, in which the corpuscles lie in the outer region of the cortex and the loop of Henle does not penetrate the medulla. The arteriole that supplies the corpuscle forms a peritubular capillary network around nephrons in the cortex

(b) Low magnification section through the kidney

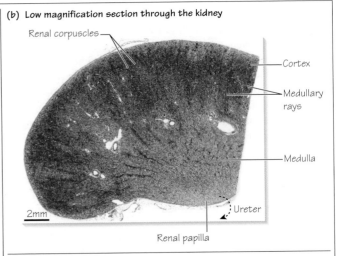

Renal corpuscles

Cortex

Medullary rays

Medulla

Ureter

Renal papilla

2mm

(c) Renal cortex

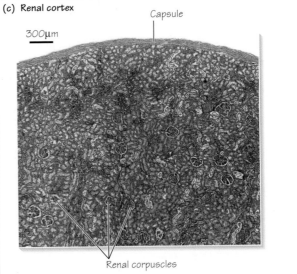

Capsule

300μm

Renal corpuscles

(d) Renal corpuscle (high magnification)

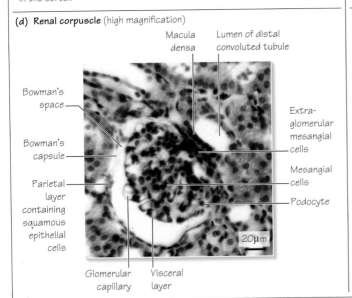

Macula densa

Lumen of distal convoluted tubule

Bowman's space

Bowman's capsule

Parietal layer containing squamous epithelial cells

Extra-glomerular mesangial cells

Mesangial cells

Podocyte

Glomerular capillary

Visceral layer

20μm

(e) Filtration

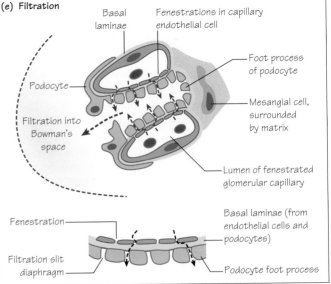

Basal laminae

Fenestrations in capillary endothelial cell

Podocyte

Filtration into Bowman's space

Foot process of podocyte

Mesangial cell, surrounded by matrix

Lumen of fenestrated glomerular capillary

Fenestration

Filtration slit diaphragm

Basal laminae (from endothelial cells and podocytes)

Podocyte foot process

The urinary system consists of two bean-shaped **kidneys** which are attached to the posterior abdominal wall, one on each side of the vertebral column. Each kidney empties into its own **ureter**, which delivers urine into a single **bladder** for storage. The bladder empties into a single **urethra**.

The kidney

The main function of the kidney is to maintain the ion balance and water content of the blood (osmoregulation) and therefore of all the other body fluids. It does this by:
• filtration of the blood;
• excretion of waste metabolic products;
• reabsorption of small molecules (glucose, amino acids, peptides), ions, and water.

In addition, the kidney regulates blood pressure and acts as an endocrine organ.

The kidney contains about 1 million functional units called **nephrons**. Filtration, excretion, and absorption take place in the nephron, and they empty into a system of collecting tubules (Fig. 32a).

The kidney contains an outer cortex and an inner medulla (Fig. 32b). These are divided up into lobes that have a pyramidal shape, in which the outer portion contains the cortex, and the inner portion, the medulla.

The cortex has a granular appearance (Fig. 32c) because it contains large numbers of ovoid filtration units (**renal corpuscles**).

The medulla has a striated appearance, because it is full of ducts and tubules, and does not contain any renal corpuscles.

The kidney has a tough outer fibrous capsule (Fig. 32c), which is made up of irregular dense connective tissue for protection. There is very little connective tissue within the kidney itself.

Nephrons

The **nephron** consists of the **renal corpuscle** and the **renal tubule** (Fig. 32a). The renal tubule is divided up into the proximal convoluted tubule (PCT), the loop of Henle, and the distal convoluted tubule (DCT) (see Chapter 33).

Renal corpuscle

The 'blind' ending of the proximal region of the nephron encapsulates a mass of **glomerular capillaries** to form the **renal corpuscle**. These are seen as ovoid structures in the cortex (Fig. 32c,d). Blood is filtered by the renal corpuscles.

Bowman's capsule encapsulates the corpuscle (Fig. 32d). It consists of an outer layer of squamous epithelium (the **parietal layer**) and an inner (visceral) layer of epithelium that contains specialized cells called **podocytes**.

Blood both enters and leaves the corpuscle via arterioles. Smooth muscle cells lining the afferent and efferent arterioles maintain a relatively high pressure along the length of the glomerular capillaries. This facilitates filtration of the blood plasma across fenestrations in the capillaries, through the basal lamina, and between the foot processes of the podocytes into Bowman's space.

Filtration occurs (Fig. 32e) due to the following structure.
• **Fenestrations** (pores) in the glomerular capillaries, 50–100 nm wide.
• The **thick basement membrane** of the capillaries, and adjacent epithelial cells. This contains a negatively charged proteoglycan (heparan sulfate), which restricts the sizes of proteins that can move across it (70 kDa or less). It also prevents positively charged proteins (e.g., albumin) from passing across, due to its negative charge.
• **Filtration slits**, 20–30 nm wide, produced by the visceral epithelial cells (**podocytes**). Podocytes project many branching 'foot' processes onto the basement membrane, which interdigitate with those from other podocytes to form the filtration slits.

The relatively high pressure in the capillaries, and their fenestrated structure, generates large quantities of glomerular filtrate. This passes out of Bowman's space into the renal tubule.

Mesangial cells, found between capillaries, are similar to pericytes and are both contractile and phagocytic. They provide support for the capillaries, turnover the basal lamina, and help to regulate blood flow in the corpuscle.

Juxtaglomerular apparatus

The **juxtaglomerular apparatus** is found next to the renal corpuscles, and it contains the **macula densa**, **juxtaglomerular cells**, and extraglomerular **mesangial** cells.
• The **macula densa** contains specialized epithelial cells in the initial portion of the DCT adjacent to the renal corpuscle. They are narrower, and their nuclei are closely spaced (Fig. 31d). They monitor the concentration of sodium and chloride ions in the filtrate, and effect release of renin by the **juxtaglomerular cells**.
• **Juxtaglomerular cells** are modified smooth muscle cells in the afferent arteriole. They monitor blood pressure and secrete renin, which converts circulating blood angiotensinogen to angiotensin I. Angiotensin I is converted to angiotensin II by angiotensin-converting enzyme (ACE).
• Angiotensin II increases smooth muscle contractility, which constricts blood vessels and thereby increases blood pressure.
• Special stains are needed to identify the juxtaglomerular cells.

33

Renal tubule

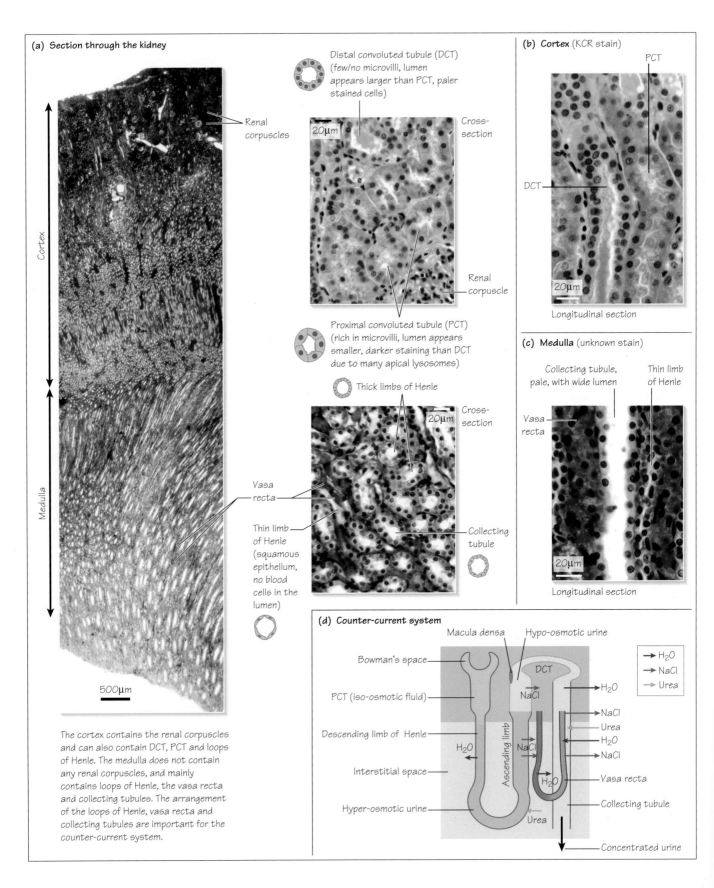

(a) Section through the kidney

Renal corpuscles

Cortex

Medulla

500μm

The cortex contains the renal corpuscles and can also contain DCT, PCT and loops of Henle. The medulla does not contain any renal corpuscles, and mainly contains loops of Henle, the vasa recta and collecting tubules. The arrangement of the loops of Henle, vasa recta and collecting tubules are important for the counter-current system.

Distal convoluted tubule (DCT) (few/no microvilli, lumen appears larger than PCT, paler stained cells)

20μm

Cross-section

Renal corpuscle

Proximal convoluted tubule (PCT) (rich in microvilli, lumen appears smaller, darker staining than DCT due to many apical lysosomes)

Thick limbs of Henle

20μm

Cross-section

Vasa recta

Thin limb of Henle (squamous epithelium, no blood cells in the lumen)

Collecting tubule

(b) Cortex (KCR stain)

PCT

DCT

20μm

Longitudinal section

(c) Medulla (unknown stain)

Collecting tubule, pale, with wide lumen

Thin limb of Henle

Vasa recta

20μm

Longitudinal section

(d) Counter-current system

Macula densa

Hypo-osmotic urine

Bowman's space

DCT

PCT (iso-osmotic fluid)

NaCl

H₂O

Descending limb of Henle

NaCl

Urea

H₂O

Ascending limb

NaCl

NaCl

Interstitial space

H₂O

Vasa recta

Hyper-osmotic urine

Collecting tubule

Urea

Concentrated urine

→ H₂O
→ NaCl
→ Urea

Once the ultrafiltrate leaves the renal corpuscle, it moves out of Bowman's space and through the renal tubule (which moves down out of the cortex, into the medulla, and then back up into the cortex, Fig. 33a,d) as described below.

Proximal convoluted tubule

The proximal convoluted tubule (PCT) is the longest part of the renal tubule and is only found in the **renal cortex**.
- It is lined by a **simple cuboidal epithelium** with a brush border (**microvilli**), which increases the surface area of these absorptive cells (Fig. 33b). The epithelium almost fills the lumen.
- Cells lining the PCT stain strongly with eosin due to their high mitochondrial and vesicular (mostly lysosomal) content. The lysosomes are important for breaking down endocytosed proteins into amino acids. Tight junctions and adherens junctions connect the cells together.
- The basal surface of the cells is highly folded, and mitochondria are packed between the folds. The mitochondria are important for providing ATP for active transport of glucose and ions.

The PCT resorbs about 80% of water (from about 150 L of fluid per day), Na^+ and Cl^-, HCO_3^- and all the proteins, amino acids and glucose from the ultrafiltrate.

The PCT cells actively transport glucose and sodium ions from the ultrafiltrate in the lumen into the interstitial tissues, and capillaries. This results in an osmotic gradient across the PCT. Chloride ions move passively out of the lumen into the PCT cells with sodium ions.

As a result of the osmotic gradient, water moves freely out of the lumen of the tubule, across the tight junctions, into the intercellular spaces between the PCT cells and then into the surrounding capillaries by osmosis. Water can also move through aquaporin channels in the cell membrane.

The ultrafiltrate in the PCT is **iso-osmotic** to blood plasma, as water and salts are resorbed in equimolar concentrations. The hormone angiotensin I stimulates water and NaCl absorption by the PCT.

Loop of Henle

This structure is mostly found in the renal medulla. It has several portions (or limbs): a thick descending portion (pars recta, or proximal straight tubule), followed by a thin descending portion, a thin ascending portion, and finally a thick ascending portion (or distal straight tubule).

The length of the thin segment is shorter in cortical nephrons than in juxtamedullary nephrons.
- A **simple thin cuboidal epithelium** lines the thick ascending and descending portions (Fig. 33c), and a **simple squamous epithelium** lines the thin portions.
- Thin segments can be distinguished from adjacent capillaries, as they do not contain blood cells in their lumens (Fig. 33c).
- The long loops of Henle and the collecting tubules are arranged in parallel to each other and to the nearby blood vessels (**vasa recta**).

The properties of the ascending and descending limbs of the loops of Henle cause the surrounding tissues (interstitium) to become hyper-osmotic with respect to blood plasma, via the countercurrent mechanism.

The **ascending limb** is permeable to NaCl and urea but not to water. Salts absorbed in this region pass into the interstitial tissue

and then into the nearby blood vessels (**vasa recta**), which make the interstitium hyper-osmotic to blood plasma.

The fluid in the **descending limb** becomes **hyper-osmotic,** as the limb descends deeper into the medulla. This is because the descending limb is permeable to water, and water moves out by osmosis, as the surrounding interstitial fluid is hyper-osmotic (Fig. 33d).

The fluid in the ascending limb becomes **hypo-osmotic** as it moves upwards. This is because as the lining cells absorb NaCl (by active transport), but not water, the overall salt content **reduces** (Fig. 33d).

The hyper-osmotic nature of the interstitium is also partly generated by the diffusion of urea, absorbed by the collecting tubules, into the interstitial space around the ascending limb.

The **vasa recta** (Fig. 33c) are derived from the efferent arterioles of the renal corpuscles, which descend into the medulla as capillaries, and then turn around and ascend into the cortex as veins, and their parallel organization to the tubules helps to maintain the hyper-osmotic gradient in interstitial tissue of the medulla.

Diuretics inhibit Na^+ absorption by the ascending limb, resulting in more dilute urine.

Distal convoluted tubule

The distal convoluted tubule (DCT) is the final short (5mm) segment of the nephron and it is found in the renal cortex (Fig. 33b).
- It stains less strongly than adjacent PCTs as it contains fewer vesicles and mitochondria.
- The lining cuboidal epithelium has fewer microvilli, and the lumen appears larger.

Less resorption occurs in the DCT compared to the PCT. Fluid entering the DCT is **hypo-osmotic** with respect to blood plasma. The DCT is impermeable to urea.

The DCT close to the renal corpuscle contains the **macula densa**, which monitors local NaCl concentration (see Chapter 32). If the **NaCl** content **drops**, it secretes high levels of the hormone **renin** (and vice versa). Renin results in the production of angiotensin II (see Chapter 32). In addition to increasing blood pressure, angiotensin II stimulates secretion of the pituitary hormone **vasopressin** (ADH or antidiuretic hormone), and the adrenal hormone **aldosterone**. Aldosterone increases uptake of NaCl from the collecting tubule. Vasopressin increases the permeability of the DCT and the cortical portions of the collecting tubules to water, concentrating urine.

Collecting tubules

Fluid from the DCT empties out into the **collecting tubules** (in the medulla), which are not part of the nephron.

A **cuboidal/columnar epithelium** lines these tubules, their lumens are large, and the epithelium is stained a pale pink (Fig. 33c). They contain principal cells (which resorb sodium ions and water, and secrete potassium ions) and intercalated cells (which secrete either hydrogen or bicarbonate ions, to regulate the acid–base balance).

Urine entering the collecting tubules is **hypo-osmotic**. The collecting tubules resorb water and NaCl from the fluid in the lumen. Urea from the interstitial spaces enters the collecting ducts. Collecting tubules empty into the ureter.

34

Ureter, urethra, and bladder

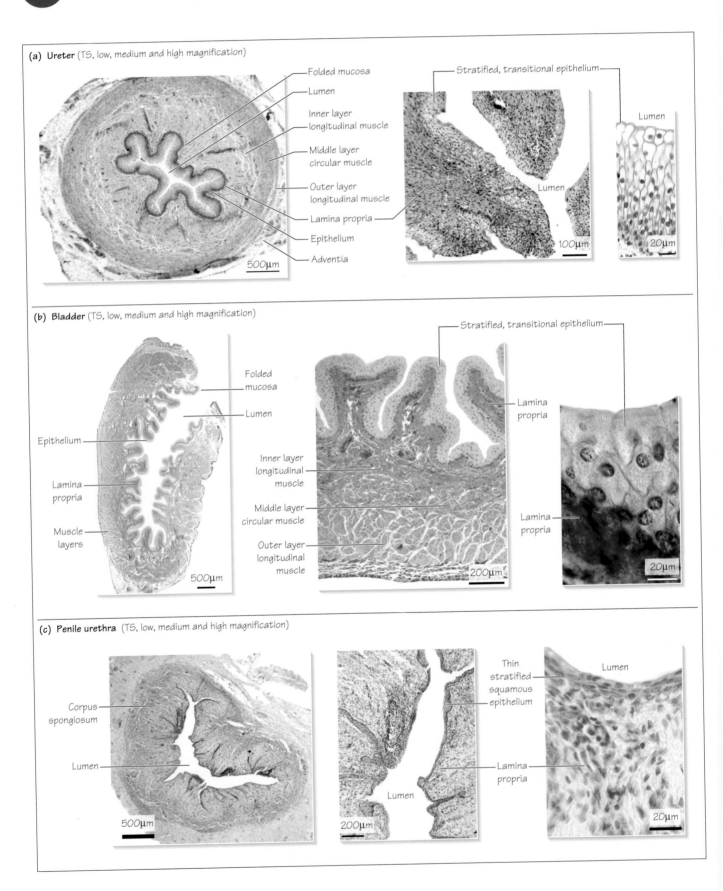

(a) Ureter (TS, low, medium and high magnification)

- Folded mucosa
- Lumen
- Inner layer longitudinal muscle
- Middle layer circular muscle
- Outer layer longitudinal muscle
- Lamina propria
- Epithelium
- Adventia

Stratified, transitional epithelium

Lumen

Lumen

500µm   100µm   20µm

(b) Bladder (TS, low, medium and high magnification)

Stratified, transitional epithelium

- Folded mucosa
- Lumen
- Epithelium
- Lamina propria
- Muscle layers

- Inner layer longitudinal muscle
- Middle layer circular muscle
- Outer layer longitudinal muscle

Lamina propria

Lamina propria

500µm   200µm   20µm

(c) Penile urethra (TS, low, medium and high magnification)

- Corpus spongiosum
- Lumen

Thin stratified squamous epithelium

Lumen

Lumen

Lamina propria

500µm   200µm   20µm

Ureter

Collecting ducts empty into the papillary ducts, and then into the **ureters** (one per kidney).

The **ureter** is a long, straight, muscle-walled tube (Fig. 34a), lined by a protective mucosa consisting of a stratified, transitional epithelium, and underlying thick, fibro-elastic lamina propria. There are no mucosal or submucosal glands, and **no submucosa**.

There is a layer of smooth muscle outside the mucosa. The upper two-thirds has **two** layers of smooth muscle. The inner layer is arranged longitudinally, and the outer is arranged circularly. The lower third has **three** layers of smooth muscle, of which the inner layer is longitudinal, the middle layer is circular, and the outer is again longitudinal.

Urine is squeezed into the bladder by peristalsis.

The outer adventitial layer consists of fibro-elastic connective tissue, and contains blood vessels, lymphatics, and nerves.

The mucosa is folded, which helps to protect against a reflux of urine when the bladder is full. (The folds are known as 'rugae'.)

Bladder

The bladder has three layers of smooth muscle, and a **transitional epithelium** (Fig. 34b). It is harder to make out the three layers, because the bladder is sac-like, not a tube, and the smooth muscle cells are more randomly organized, forming a syncytium.

The mucosa is heavily folded. This helps the bladder accommodate large volume changes between an empty and full bladder.

As the bladder enlarges, when it fills with urine, the transitional epithelial lining can stretch until it looks like stratified squamous epithelium.

The epithelial lining forms an impermeable barrier against urine.

Urethra

The urethra (Fig. 34c) conveys urine from the bladder to the exterior of the body. It is similar in structure to the ureter, though shorter.

In males, the urethra is about 20 cm long, and is divided into three sections: the prostatic (receives ejaculatory ducts and ducts of the prostate), membranous, and penile (receives the ducts of the bulbourethral glands).

The epithelium gradually changes from **transitional** to pseudostratified columnar and finally to **stratified squamous epithelium**, distally, as shown here.

Its lumen is kept closed, unless urine is being passed.

In females, the urethra is much shorter (about 5 cm). It is lined by a **stratified squamous epithelium** and is surrounded by an internal layer of smooth muscle, and an outer layer of striated muscle.

The mucosa of the female urethra contains mucous-secreting glands, which lubricate the lining, facilitating the passage of urine.

The female urethra is attached to the anterior wall of the vagina by an external layer of fibrous connective tissue.

The shortness of the female urethra contributes to the high frequency of urinary tract infections in women, every year affecting about 20% of women between the ages of 20 and 56 years. About half of all women will experience a urinary tract infection during their lifetime. A common cause of infection is sexual intercourse, which probably results in mechanical transfer of bacteria into the urethra, which can then travel up towards the bladder.

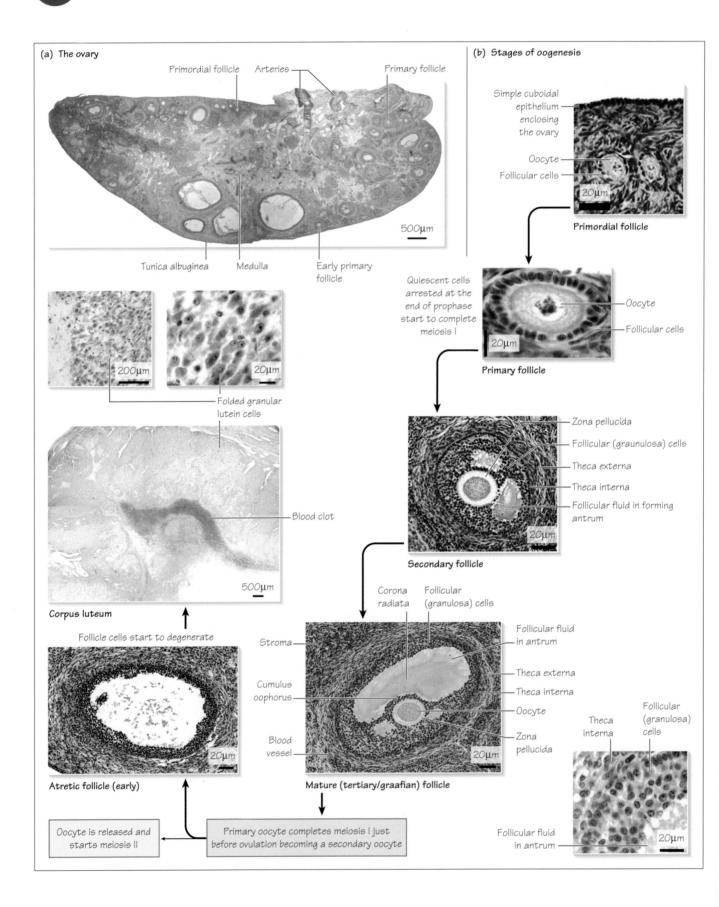

(a) The ovary

Primordial follicle · Arteries · Primary follicle

500μm

Tunica albuginea · Medulla · Early primary follicle

200μm

20μm

Folded granular lutein cells

Blood clot

500μm

Corpus luteum

Follicle cells start to degenerate

20μm

Atretic follicle (early)

Oocyte is released and starts meiosis II

Primary oocyte completes meiosis I just before ovulation becoming a secondary oocyte

(b) Stages of oogenesis

Simple cuboidal epithelium enclosing the ovary

Oocyte

Follicular cells

20μm

Primordial follicle

Quiescent cells arrested at the end of prophase start to complete meiosis I

Oocyte

Follicular cells

20μm

Primary follicle

Zona pellucida

Follicular (graunulosa) cells

Theca externa

Theca interna

Follicular fluid in forming antrum

20μm

Secondary follicle

Corona radiata · Follicular (granulosa) cells

Stroma

Cumulus oophorus

Blood vessel

Follicular fluid in antrum

Theca externa

Theca interna

Oocyte

Zona pellucida

20μm

Mature (tertiary/graafian) follicle

Theca interna · Follicular (granulosa) cells

Follicular fluid in antrum

20μm

The ovary

The pair of ovaries mature and release eggs (oogenesis), and produce and secrete hormones. The ovaries are covered by a tunica albuginea, which consists of a simple cuboidal epithelium, with underlying fine collagen fibers in a parallel organization together with spindle-shaped cells (Fig. 35a). Ovarian follicles are found in the cortex. The medulla is a highly vascular medulla, containing coiled (helicine) arteries.

Oogenesis

In early embryogenesis, primordial germ cells from the yolk sac (extra-embryonic) migrate into the developing gonad, where they differentiate into oogonia, and proliferate.

Between 3 and 8 months of gestation, oogonia enlarge and develop into primary oocytes, which begin meiosis but become arrested in the last stage of prophase in the first meiotic division, forming primordial follicles.

Primordial follicles

These contain a single layer of flattened **ovarian follicular epithelial cells** (granulosa cells) around the oocyte (Fig. 35b). They are small, and usually found close to the outer edge of the cortex. At birth, the ovary contains around 400 000 primordial follicles, and no further follicles develop after birth.

At the onset of puberty, pituitary hormones, follicle-stimulating hormone (FSH) and luteinizing hormone (LH), start monthly (menstrual) cycles of egg production.

Primary follicles

At the start of each menstrual cycle, FSH stimulates 12–20 primordial follicles (Fig. 35b) to develop into primary follicles.
• The layer of follicular cells surrounding the oocyte proliferates to form two layers (**zona granulosa**).
• The primary oocyte re-enters meiosis I.
• A thick glycoprotein layer, the **zona pellucida**, develops around the oocyte.
• The **stroma** (connective tissue) around the follicle develops to form a capsule-like 'theca', which differentiates into two layers: the **theca interna** (rounded cells that secrete androgens and follicular fluid) and a more fibrous **theca externa** (spindle-shaped cells that do not secrete androgens).

Secondary follicles

The primary follicle develops into a **secondary follicle**, in which the follicular cells have proliferated and enlarged (Fig. 35b). Small areas of nutritive fluid (follicular fluid) secreted by the follicular cells have accumulated in the intracellular spaces. These gradually coalesce to form an **antrum** in the tertiary follicle.

Tertiary/graafian follicles

Characteristics of this type of follicle (Fig. 35b):
• The follicular fluid fills a single space, the **antrum**, which is surrounded by an outer layer of follicular cells (**membrana granulosa**).

• The granulosa cells that directly surround the oocyte, and project into the antrum are called the **corona radiata**.
• A layer of granulosa cells between the corona radiata and the theca interna are called the **cumulus oophorus**.
• There is a basement membrane between the granulosa cells and the **theca interna**.
• The fibrous **theca externa** merges with the surrounding stroma.

Follicular cell expansion results in a rise in estrogen, as these cells convert androgens into estrogen, and secrete it. Negative feedback to the pituitary gland lowers the level of FSH. The follicular cells also release inhibin, which lowers FSH. The increased estrogen level results in LH release. LH induces connections between follicular cells to loosen, facilitating the release of the oocyte.

The primary oocyte completes its first meiotic division in the **tertiary/graafian follicle** shortly before ovulation. Only one secondary oocyte is observed, because most of the cytoplasm goes into one of the two daughter cells, while the other disintegrates into a small polar body, which is difficult to see.

The **oocyte, zona pellucida**, and **corona radiata** are all expelled at ovulation, and enter the fallopian tube.

The oocyte then begins its second meiotic division, becoming arrested in metaphase II. Division only continues if the ovum is fertilized. Again one of the two daughter cells receives all the cytoplasm, and the other forms the degenerate polar body. Ruptured follicles collapse and fill with a blood clot (corpus haemorrhagicum), and then luteinize, forming a transitory endocrine organ called the **corpus luteum** (LH induced).

Corpus luteum

In the corpus luteum (Fig. 35b), the granulosa cells enlarge, become vesicular, and develop into **granulosa lutein** cells. **Theca interna** cells invade the spaces between these cells and they also enlarge and develop into glandular **theca lutein** cells. The pigmented lutein cells can make the corpus luteum appear yellow.

The **granulosa lutein** cells secrete progesterone.

The corpus luteum also secretes estrogen (which inhibits FSH) and relaxin (which relaxes the fibro-cartilage of the pubic symphysis).

Increased progesterone levels suppress further release of LH by the pituitary gland.

The corpus luteum develops into a large structure, up to 5 cm in humans.

If fertilization does not occur, the corpus luteum degenerates into a small white fibrous scar (**corpus albicans**). The subsequent decline in **progesterone** levels precipitates **menstruation**.

Decreased estrogen levels also help to precipitate menstruation, and increase FSH secretion.

If pregnancy occurs, then the syncytiotrophoblasts of the placenta release **human chorionic gonadotropin** and the corpus luteum persists.

Only one of the maturing follicles completes the maturation process each month, with the remainder degenerating into **atretic** follicles. Follicular maturation takes about 3 months.

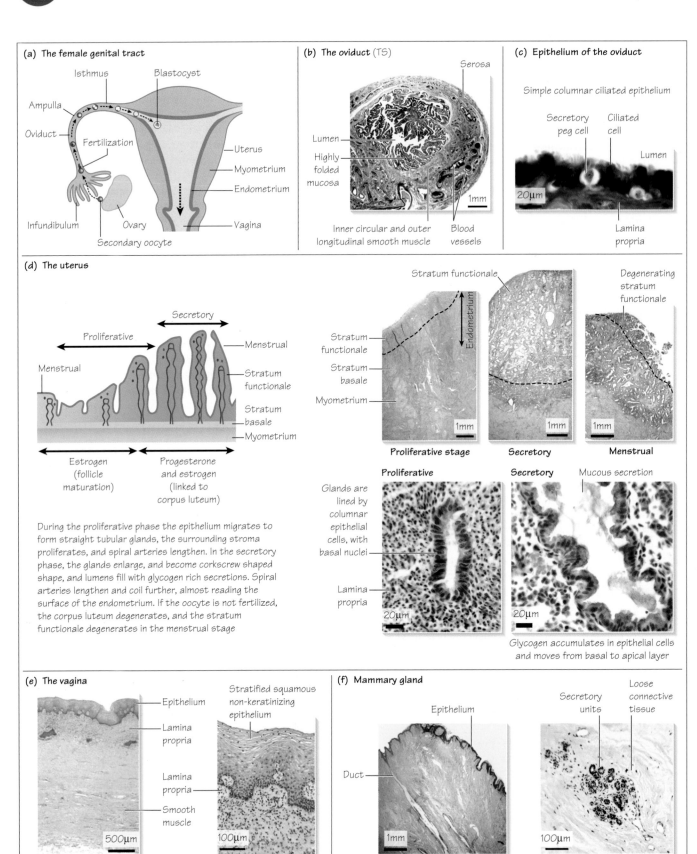

(a) The female genital tract

Isthmus

Blastocyst

Ampulla

Oviduct

Fertilization

Infundibulum

Secondary oocyte

Ovary

Uterus

Myometrium

Endometrium

Vagina

(b) The oviduct (TS)

Serosa

Lumen

Highly folded mucosa

1mm

Inner circular and outer longitudinal smooth muscle

Blood vessels

(c) Epithelium of the oviduct

Simple columnar ciliated epithelium

Secretory peg cell

Ciliated cell

Lumen

20μm

Lamina propria

(d) The uterus

Secretory

Proliferative

Menstrual

Menstrual

Stratum functionale

Stratum basale

Myometrium

Estrogen (follicle maturation)

Progesterone and estrogen (linked to corpus luteum)

During the proliferative phase the epithelium migrates to form straight tubular glands, the surrounding stroma proliferates, and spiral arteries lengthen. In the secretory phase, the glands enlarge, and become corkscrew shaped shape, and lumens fill with glycogen rich secretions. Spiral arteries lengthen and coil further, almost reading the surface of the endometrium. If the oocyte is not fertilized, the corpus luteum degenerates, and the stratum functionale degenerates in the menstrual stage

Stratum functionale

Stratum functionale

Degenerating stratum functionale

Stratum functionale

Stratum basale

Myometrium

Endometrium

1mm

1mm

1mm

Proliferative stage

Secretory

Menstrual

Proliferative

Secretory

Mucous secretion

Glands are lined by columnar epithelial cells, with basal nuclei

Lamina propria

20μm

20μm

Glycogen accumulates in epithelial cells and moves from basal to apical layer

(e) The vagina

Epithelium

Lamina propria

Lamina propria

Smooth muscle

Stratified squamous non-keratinizing epithelium

500μm

100μm

(f) Mammary gland

Epithelium

Duct

Secretory units

Loose connective tissue

1mm

100μm

The female genital tract consists of the oviduct (or fallopian tubes), the uterus, and the vagina, making up the rest of the female reproductive system (Fig. 36a). The oviducts transport the ova to the uterus. The uterus is a muscular organ, and its mucosal lining undergoes hormone-dependent changes. The vagina is a muscular tube that leads to the exterior of the body.

The fallopian tube/oviduct

The released ovum enters into the flared and 'fringed' (fimbriated) **proximal** region (**infundibulum**) of the oviduct (Fig. 36a), then moves into a longer, thin-walled **ampulla**, followed by a short thicker-walled **isthmus**. This leads into an **intramural portion**, which extends through the uterine wall, and opens into the uterine lumen. The ovum is fertilized in the oviduct.

The mucosa has primary, secondary and tertiary longitudinal folds, giving it a labyrinthine appearance (Fig. 36b).

The **muscularis mucosa** contains an outer longitudinal and inner circular layer, which gently contracts to propel the ovum towards the uterus, and is surrounded by an outer layer of loose supporting tissue (serosa). The isthmus has fewer longitudinal mucosal folds.

The epithelium (Fig. 36c) contains the following types of cell.
• **Peg cells:** non-ciliated columnar cells (P). They are secretory and have extensive Golgi. They secrete nutrient material into the lumen, to support the ovum. Peg cells are particularly well developed and easy to see at day 14 of the menstrual cycle, around the time of ovulation.
• **Ciliated cells:** ciliated columnar cells. Some cells have large accumulations of glycogen. The cilia help to move the fluid away from the ovary towards the uterus, thus moving the ovum towards the uterus.
• **Intercalated cells:** possibly a morphological variant of secretory cells.

The uterus

The uterus is made up of an external layer of smooth muscle (**myometrium**) and an internal layer (**endometrium**). The central layer of the myometrium is rich in large blood vessels and lymphatics, and is surrounded by smooth muscle bundles in the inner and outer layers.

The **endometrium** has two layers, the **inner stratum basale** layer, and the **outer stratum functionale** layer (Fig. 36d). During the menstrual cycle, the endometrium changes its appearance, and its thickness increases from 1 mm just after menstruation to about 6 mm in the 'secretory' phase (Fig. 36d).

Proliferative phase (first half of the menstrual cycle)

• The **stratum functionale** layer proliferates. The surface epithelium invaginates to form tubular (**endometrial**) glands in the underlying lamina propria (**endometrial stroma**). The glands open out onto the surface.
• The connective tissue in the stroma also proliferates.
• Radial arteries (branches from the uterine artery) enter the basal layer of the endometrium, where they branch into small straight arteries, and also continue as highly coiled 'spiral' arteries, which supply a rich capillary bed in the endometrium.

Secretory phase (after ovulation)

The secretory phase begins after ovulation (Fig. 36d), as the corpus luteum becomes active. In this phase, the endometrial glands become corkscrew-shaped, fill with glycogen, and secrete a glycogen-rich secretion.

Menstrual phase

If the ovum is not fertilized, the corpus luteum degenerates, and the decrease in estrogen and progesterone levels results in the constriction of **spiral arterioles** in the **stratum functionalis** layer. This is followed by **ischemia**, and the degeneration of the functionalis layer. The arteries rupture, and the rapid blood flow dislodges the necrotic functionale layer, which is lost. About 35–50 mL of blood is lost over 5 days.

The vagina

The vagina is a muscular tube (Fig. 36e), which has a protective thick **stratified squamous epithelium**. The underlying layer of **lamina propria** is rich in elastic fibers, and does not have any glands.

A layer of **smooth muscle**, which has an inner circular and outer longitudinal layer, lies underneath the lamina propria.

The outer adventitial layer merges with that of the bladder (anteriorly) and rectum (posteriorly).

The elastic lamina propria and the layer of smooth muscle enable the vagina to distend, particularly during childbirth.

The vagina is lubricated by **cervical mucus**, which is derived from the rich vascular network, and mucus from tall columnar mucous secretory cells in the endocervical canal.

The smooth muscle contracts during and after coitus to keep the pool of semen close to the cervix. It also plays a role in childbirth, allowing the vagina to distend.

Mammary glands

Each breast is made up of 15–25 secretory lobes, embedded in adipose tissue.

The mammary gland is similar to a modified sweat gland (Fig. 36f). Each secretory lobe is a compound tubular acinar gland.

The acini empty into ducts, which are lined by cuboidal, or low columnar epithelial cells, and surrounded by myoepithelial cells. The epithelium of these ducts proliferates during the menstrual cycle.

The ducts from each lobule empty into a lactiferous duct that empties onto the surface of the nipple. These ducts are surrounded by smooth muscle in the region of the nipple, contraction of which makes the nipple become erect.

The lumina become more prominent during the midpoint of the menstrual cycle.

In pregnant women, the alveolar duct epithelium proliferates, lots of secretory alveoli form, and they begin to make a protein-rich fluid called colostrum.

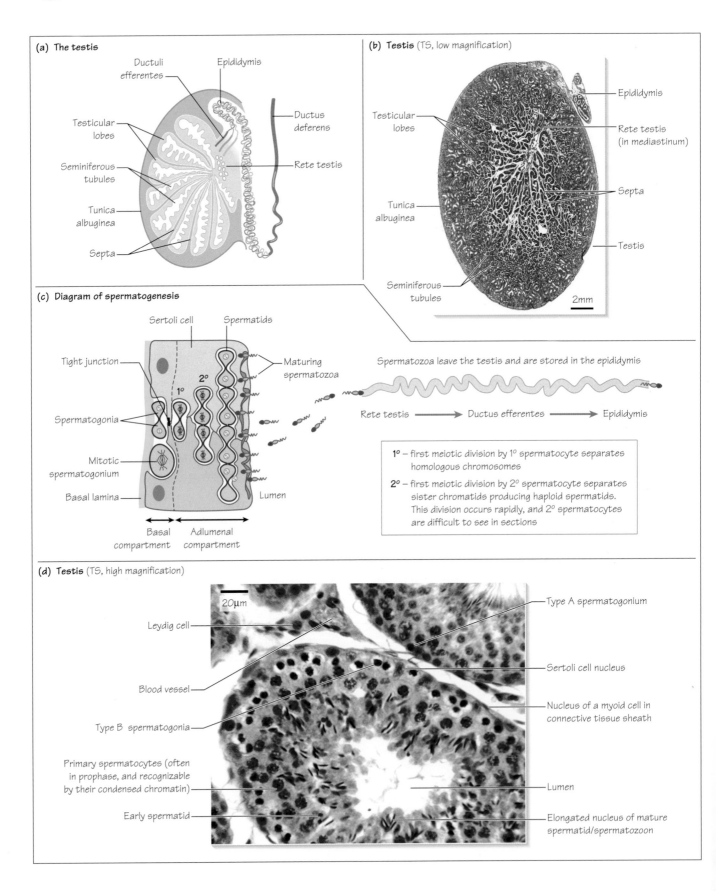

(a) The testis

Ductuli efferentes
Epididymis
Ductus deferens
Testicular lobes
Seminiferous tubules
Tunica albuginea
Septa
Rete testis

(b) Testis (TS, low magnification)

Testicular lobes
Tunica albuginea
Seminiferous tubules
Epididymis
Rete testis (in mediastinum)
Septa
Testis

2mm

(c) Diagram of spermatogenesis

Sertoli cell
Spermatids
Tight junction
Spermatogonia
Mitotic spermatogonium
Basal lamina
Maturing spermatozoa
Lumen
Basal compartment
Adlumenal compartment

Spermatozoa leave the testis and are stored in the epididymis

Rete testis → Ductus efferentes → Epididymis

1° – first meiotic division by 1° spermatocyte separates homologous chromosomes

2° – first meiotic division by 2° spermatocyte separates sister chromatids producing haploid spermatids. This division occurs rapidly, and 2° spermatocytes are difficult to see in sections

(d) Testis (TS, high magnification)

20μm

Leydig cell
Blood vessel
Type B spermatogonia
Primary spermatocytes (often in prophase, and recognizable by their condensed chromatin)
Early spermatid
Type A spermatogonium
Sertoli cell nucleus
Nucleus of a myoid cell in connective tissue sheath
Lumen
Elongated nucleus of mature spermatid/spermatozoon

The main functions of this system are to produce spermatozoa and androgens (sex hormones, principally testosterone) and to facilitate fertilization, by introducing spermatozoa into the female genital tract (copulation).

This system includes the testis, genital ducts, accessory sex glands, and penis. The pair of testes produces spermatozoa and androgens. Accessory glands produce the fluid constituents of semen. Long genital ducts store sperm and transport them to the penis.

The testis

The testis (Fig. 37a) produces male gametes (spermatozoa) and secretes male sex hormones. The **tunica albuginea** is a thick fibromuscular connective tissue capsule that surrounds the testis (Fig. 37b). Septa within the testis are formed by connective tissue emanating from the tunica albuginea, which divide it into about 250 incomplete **lobules**. The septa converge at a thickening of the tunica albuginea called the **mediastinum**, which contains the **rete testis**, a network of anastomosing tubules. Each lobule contains 1–4 **seminiferous tubules**, 30–70 cm long.

Spermatogenic cells, spermatogenesis, and spermiogenesis

Spermatogenesis (sperm formation) occurs in the seminiferous tubules (Fig. 37c,d). A complex stratified germinal (seminiferous epithelium) lines the tubules. It contains two distinct populations of cells, spermatogenic and Sertoli cells.

Four haploid gametes (mature spermatocytes) result from one **spermatogenic cell** following two meiotic divisions.

Proliferating mitotic Type B spermatogonia (pale staining) in the basal layer of the epithelium move towards the lumen of the tubule, and begin the first meiotic division. Following this division they become primary (1°) spermatocytes. Each primary spermatocyte undergoes a second (2°) meiotic division to form haploid 2° spermatocytes. These then start to shed their cytoplasm and develop into mature spermatozoa (a process called **spermiogenesis**).

During spermatogenesis, the developing cells move from the basal layer of the tubules towards the lumen.

The developing spermatozoa remain connected to each other by cytoplasmic bridges until this process is complete. It takes about 74 days to produce mature human spermatozoa from a type A spermatogenic cell. Type A spermatogonia are darkly staining, reserve stem cells found next to the basal lamina. These reserve cells replenish the type B population.

Sertoli cells

These are tall columnar cells, which extend from the basement membrane to the lumen. They form pockets around the proliferating and differentiating germ cells, transferring nutrients to them from nearby capillaries.

• Sertoli cells form an important barrier, the **blood–testis** barrier. Continuous tight junctions between these cells separate the tubules into a basal and an adluminal compartment, forming a barrier between them. The blood–testis barrier isolates the developing spermatogonia, spermatocytes, and mature spermatozoa from blood. Differentiating spermatogonia enter the **adluminal compartment**, and are sealed off from the basal compartment. If novel antigens are expressed on the haploid cells, then it is less likely that they will be detected by the immune system in this sealed-off and protective compartment.

• **Sertoli cells** phagocytose the excess spermatid cytoplasm, shed as they develop into mature spermatozoa, as well as degenerating germ cells. They aid the passage of developing spermatocytes from the basal to the adluminal layer.

• **Sertoli cells** produce and secrete **testicular fluid**, which contains a protein that binds to and concentrates **testosterone**, a hormone essential for the development of spermatozoa. Testosterone is released from pale-staining Leydig cells found between the tubules close to blood vessels.

The nuclei of **Sertoli** cells are pale with dense nucleoli and are found close to the basal lamina of the tubules (Fig. 37d).

A sheath of connective tissue, which contains **fibroblasts** and contractile **myoid cells**, surrounds the tubules (Fig. 37d). The myoid cells generate gentle peristaltic waves in the tubules.

Before puberty, the tubules only contain small numbers of primitive germ cells, which have an extra-embryonic origin (they derive from the yolk sac endoderm). After puberty (driven by testosterone) the spermatogonia multiply continuously to form male gametes.

Effects of hormones on Leydig and Sertoli cells

Secretion of testosterone by the pale-staining 'interstitial' Leydig cells, found in the tissue between the tubules (Fig. 37d), is stimulated by luteinizing hormone from the pituitary gland. Their cytoplasm is full of cholesterol-lipid droplets, which is used to make **testosterone**. Testosterone promotes production of spermatozoa, secretion from the accessory sex glands, and acquisition of male secondary characteristics.

Follicle-stimulating hormone (FSH) secreted by the pituitary stimulates the Sertoli cells to secrete androgen-binding protein into the lumen of the seminiferous tubules. Binding of testosterone in the lumen provides a local testosterone supply for the developing spermatogonia.

(a) The genital ducts

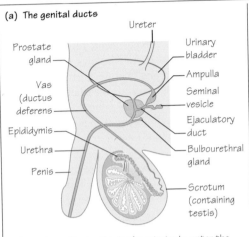

Prostate gland
Ureter
Urinary bladder
Vas (ductus deferens)
Ampulla
Seminal vesicle
Ejaculatory duct
Epididymis
Urethra
Bulbourethral gland
Penis
Scrotum (containing testis)

Sperm leave the testis via the rete tesis, enter the ductus efferentes, and then move into the epididymis, where they are stored (in the tail of the epididymis) and matured. This is a highly coiled tube, and the lumens of multiple ducts are seen in cross-section as shown here in the low magnification image

(b) Epididymis (TS, low magnification)

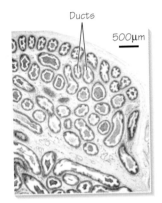

Ducts
500μm

(c) Epididymis (TS, high magnification)

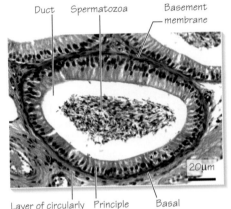

Duct   Spermatozoa   Basement membrane

20μm

Layer of circularly arranged smooth muscle
Principle (columnar) cell with long microvilli
Basal cell

The epithelium of the epididymis is pseudostratified with two major cell types: basal and principle cells

(d) Vas deferens (TS, low magnification)

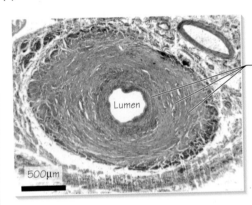

Lumen

Three layers of smooth muscle (inner and outer are longitudinal and middle layer is circular)

500μm

(e) Epithelium of vas deferens (TS, high magnification)

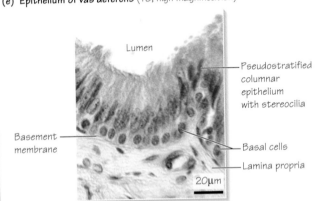

Lumen

Pseudostratified columnar epithelium with stereocilia

Basement membrane

Basal cells

Lamina propria

20μm

(f) Penis (fetal penis, TS, low magnification)

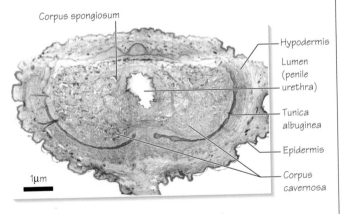

Corpus spongiosum

Hypodermis
Lumen (penile urethra)
Tunica albuginea
Epidermis
Corpus cavernosa

1μm

The two corpus cavernosa and the corpus spongionsum are cylindrical masses of errectile tissue. They contain many blood sinusoids, which fill with arterial blood during an erection

(g) Epithelium of the penis (urethra)

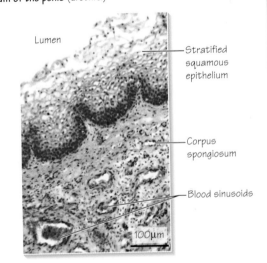

Lumen

Stratified squamous epithelium

Corpus spongiosum

Blood sinusoids

100μm

The genital ducts in the male genital tract are used for the transport of spermatozoa from the testes to the exterior of the body (Fig. 38a). The looped **seminiferous tubules** are connected to (in sequence) the **tubuli recti** (short straight tubules connected to the seminiferous tubules, with low columnar epithelium), the **rete testis** (anastomosing tubules lined by a low cuboidal epithelium), followed by the **ductuli efferentes**, which lead into the **ductus epididymus**.

The **ductus epididymus** both stores and matures spermatozoa, so that they become competent to fertilize ova. On ejaculation they are emptied into the **ductus (vas) deferens**, and then into the **ejaculatory duct**, before passing into the **urethra** and finally to the exterior of the body.

The epididymis

The **ductuli efferentes** together with the **ductus epididymus** make up the **epididymis**. These ducts are highly coiled, and make up a single tube in the epididymis that would be up to 6 meters long if unraveled. This means that several sections of it can be found on a single slide (Fig. 38b).
• The **ductus epididymus** both stores and matures the spermatozoa, so that they become competent to fertilize ova.
• The lining epithelium is pseudostratified (Fig. 38c). It contains tall columnar lining cells (principal cells) that have long, non-motile branching microvilli (stereocilia), and basal (stem) cells, which renew the population of principal cells. The principal cells reabsorb most of the testicular fluid that was secreted by the seminiferous tubules.
• Layers of circularly arranged smooth muscle surround the ductus epididymus. Slow contractions of this muscle layer result in the movement of sperm along the duct from the start (head) to the end (tail).

Ductus (vas) deferens

This is a thick-walled tube, which is lined with an inner and outer layer of longitudinal smooth muscle and a middle layer of circular muscle (Fig. 38d).

The vas deferens is about 45 cm long and connects the epididymis to the urethra.

This muscular tube contracts when stimulated by nerves from the sympathetic nervous system, expelling its contents into the urethra during ejaculation.
• The duct is lined by a pseudostratified epithelium (Fig. 38e).
• The supporting lamina propria is folded, allowing the duct to expand during ejaculation.

A duct from the seminal vesicles (see Chapter 39) drains into the distal portion of ductus deferens (the ampulla), to form the short ejaculatory duct. These ducts converge to join the urethra, as they pass through the prostate gland.

Penis

The penis contains three cylindrical cavernous bodies (**corpora**), a pair of **corpora cavernosa**, and the **corpus spongiosum**, which surround the urethra, ending in the glans penis (Fig. 38f). Penile skin moves freely over the underlying tissues due to the loose **hypodermis**. Unless circumcised, it extends over the glans as the prepuce (foreskin) a retractable protective fold of skin.

A tough fibrous sheath or **tunica albuginea** surrounds each of the corpora.

The **corpora** contain irregular vascular spaces (sinusoids), lined by endothelium.

Erection of the penis results from relaxation of smooth muscle in the thick-walled distributing arteries, following parasympathetic stimulation and, as a result, the vascular sinusoids fill with blood. As the corpora distend, they press against the inextensible tunica albuginea, compressing the veins, so blood is less able to drain away. The penis fills with blood and becomes erect. The penile urethra is not compressed or closed because the tunica albuginea of the corpus spongiosum is more extensible than that of the other corpora.

Penile urethra

The urethra, which is 20 cm long, has three parts. The prostatic urethra is the region into which the ejaculatory ducts of the prostate gland (see Chapter 39) empty, and a transitional epithelium lines this region. This is followed by a short 'membranous urethra' and finally, the penile urethra. The ducts of the bulbourethral glands empty into this final portion, which has a protective stratified epithelium (Fig. 38g).

Accessory sex glands

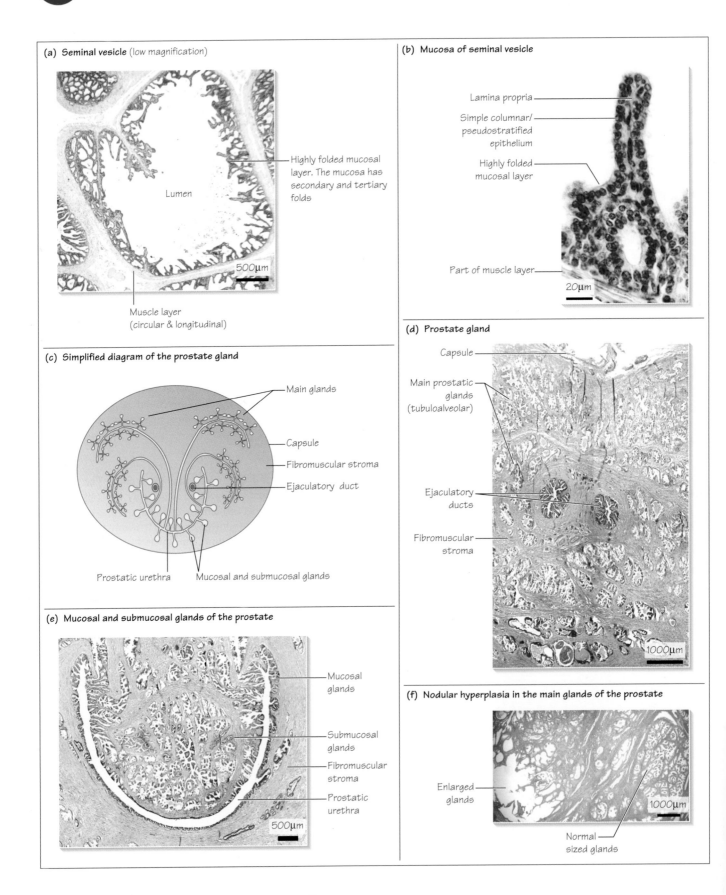

(a) **Seminal vesicle** (low magnification)

Highly folded mucosal layer. The mucosa has secondary and tertiary folds

Lumen

Muscle layer (circular & longitudinal)

500μm

(b) **Mucosa of seminal vesicle**

Lamina propria

Simple columnar/ pseudostratified epithelium

Highly folded mucosal layer

Part of muscle layer

20μm

(c) **Simplified diagram of the prostate gland**

Main glands

Capsule

Fibromuscular stroma

Ejaculatory duct

Prostatic urethra

Mucosal and submucosal glands

(d) **Prostate gland**

Capsule

Main prostatic glands (tubuloalveolar)

Ejaculatory ducts

Fibromuscular stroma

1000μm

(e) **Mucosal and submucosal glands of the prostate**

Mucosal glands

Submucosal glands

Fibromuscular stroma

Prostatic urethra

500μm

(f) **Nodular hyperplasia in the main glands of the prostate**

Enlarged glands

Normal sized glands

1000μm

The **seminal vesicles** and **prostate glands** both empty their secretions into the prostate region of the urethra, and are responsible for producing most of the seminal fluid. In addition, there are also the bulbourethral glands of Cowper (not shown here). This gland secretes galactose and sialic acid into the penile urethra, just prior to ejaculation, to lubricate the epithelial surface of the urethra.

Seminal vesicles

The seminal vesicles secrete a viscous fluid that is rich in fructose, the major source of energy for the ejaculated sperm. There are two seminal vesicles, and together, they secrete up to 85% of the total volume of seminal fluid. They deliver this fluid via a duct into the ductus deferens as it penetrates the prostate gland, in a short region known as the ejaculatory duct.

The seminal vesicles consist of an outer layer of connective tissue (Fig. 39a), two layers of smooth muscle, of which the inner layer is circularly arranged and the outer longitudinally. The innermost layer is made up of a highly folded mucosa.

The lumen of each vesicle is highly irregular because the mucosa is highly folded. This gives the lumen a honeycomb appearance at low magnification.
• The lining epithelium is **pseudostratified tall columnar epithelium** (Fig. 39b).
• The secretory cells have a prominent Golgi apparatus, and stain palely due to the large amounts of secretory vesicles containing lipid droplets in the cytoplasm.
• The secreted fluid is yellow, viscid, and alkaline. It contains fructose, fibrinogen, vitamin C, and prostaglandins. Fructose is used as the main energy source by the ejaculated sperm.

During ejaculation, sympathetic stimulation causes contraction of the smooth muscle, forcing the secreted fluid into the urethra.

Prostate gland

The prostate gland (Fig. 39c) is the largest of the three accessory sex glands, and actually consists of many (up to 50) glands. The outer peripheral region of the prostate contains the main glands (peripheral compound glands; Fig. 39d). The inner region contains **mucosal** and **submucosal** glands (Fig. 39e). All of these glands secrete their contents into excretory ducts that empty into the prostatic urethra, in the central region of the gland.

The glands are branched (compound glands), and lined by a **simple/pseudostratified columnar epithelium**, which is highly folded.

The epithelium is supported by a fibro-elastic lamina propria.

The glands secrete a thin and milky secretion, which is rich in citric acid, and hydrolytic enzymes, including fibrinolysin.

These enzymes liquefy coagulated semen after it has been deposited in the female genital tract.

The secretory units are surrounded by a fibromuscular stroma that contracts to expel the secretions during ejaculation.

The mucosal and submucosal glands within the prostate gland can enlarge with age (benign hyperplasia; Fig. 39f), which can cause problems with urination.

The main glands can become transformed, resulting in prostate cancer. Male sex hormones (androgens) are implicated in both cases, and one form of treatment is to remove the testes, thus removing the source of androgens.

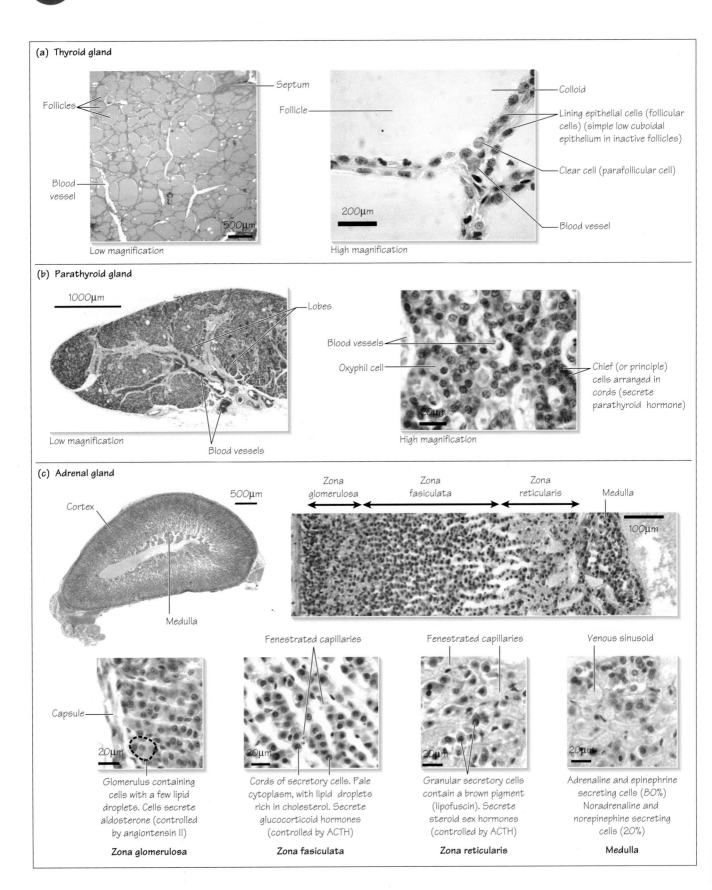

(a) Thyroid gland

Follicles

Septum

Follicle

Colloid

Lining epithelial cells (follicular cells) (simple low cuboidal epithelium in inactive follicles)

Clear cell (parafollicular cell)

Blood vessel

Blood vessel

500µm

200µm

Low magnification

High magnification

(b) Parathyroid gland

1000µm

Lobes

Blood vessels

Oxyphil cell

Chief (or principle) cells arranged in cords (secrete parathyroid hormone)

Low magnification

Blood vessels

20µm

High magnification

(c) Adrenal gland

Cortex

Medulla

Zona glomerulosa

Zona fasiculata

Zona reticularis

Medulla

500µm

100µm

Medulla

Fenestrated capillaries

Fenestrated capillaries

Venous sinusoid

Capsule

20µm

20µm

20µm

20µm

Glomerulus containing cells with a few lipid droplets. Cells secrete aldosterone (controlled by angiontensin II)

Cords of secretory cells. Pale cytoplasm, with lipid droplets rich in cholesterol. Secrete glucocorticoid hormones (controlled by ACTH)

Granular secretory cells contain a brown pigment (lipofuscin). Secrete steroid sex hormones (controlled by ACTH)

Adrenaline and epinephrine secreting cells (80%) Noradrenaline and norepinephine secreting cells (20%)

Zona glomerulosa

Zona fasiculata

Zona reticularis

Medulla

Definition: A gland is an **organized collection** of **secretory epithelial cells**.

Exocrine glands deliver their secretions onto the surface of epithelia via ducts (see Chapters 7 and 28).

Endocrine glands secrete hormones directly into the bloodstream, do not have ducts, and are supplied by a rich network of blood vessels.

Hormones can act **directly** on non-endocrine tissues, or **indirectly** modulate the secretory activity of other glands.

Hormones are derived from **cholesterol** (steroid hormones, lipid-soluble) **peptide**/protein or glycoprotein hormones, or modified amino acids (catecholamines, bind to receptors in plasma membrane of target cells).

Secretions can be:
• **paracrine:** hormones act on nearby tissues and cells; or
• **neuroendocrine:** hormones travel long distances through the blood to act on a specific 'target' organ, analogous to the co-ordinating activity of neurons.

Endocrine glands can be:
• **a component of a gland with both endocrine and exocrine functions** (e.g., kidney, pancreas, and gonads);
• **a discrete endocrine gland**, that only has endocrine function, such as the pituitary (hypophysis), thyroid, parathyroid, adrenal, and pineal glands;
• **a diffuse neuroendocrine system** (e.g., cells in the gut, which secrete low molecular-weight peptides such as cholecystokinin and secretin).

Thyroid gland

The thyroid gland is located in the neck, and contains two lobes (about 5 cm × 2.5 cm). It contains many thyroid follicles, which store colloid (Fig. 40a). Colloid is an inactive precursor of thyroid hormone bound to a glycoprotein (thyroglobulin). Follicles are cavities surrounded by epithelial cells (follicular cells), which secrete the hormone.

To secrete active hormone, lining epithelial cells engulf the colloid, use hydrolytic enzymes to break it down, and then release active hormone into the blood. Active follicular cells are columnar.

The two hormones secreted (**thyroxine** or T4 and the more active **tri-iodothyronine** or T3) regulate the basal metabolic rate. The pituitary hormone, thyroid-stimulating hormone (TSH), regulates their release by indirect action.

The lining epithelium also contains parafollicular (clear) cells (Fig. 40a). These cells secrete **calcitonin**, which regulates blood calcium levels. Parafollicular cells are scattered among the follicular cells, and while they can be recognized from their pale cytoplasm, they are difficult to identify with light microscopy.

In **hyperthyroidism**, the thyroid becomes enlarged and hyperactive, and the follicles look smaller.

Parathyroid glands

These consist of a pair of ovoid glands associated with the thyroid. Each gland is divided into lobules by connective tissue septa (Fig. 40b).

The parathyroid contains two types of cells (Fig. 40b). **Chief (or principal) cells** are small and pale, weakly eosinophilic staining, and contain cytoplasmic granules. They secrete parathyroid hormone (PTH). About 80% of the cells are inactive and have paler cytoplasm than active cells. PTH acts on the epithelial cells in the kidney (renal tubule) and osteoclasts in bone to raise Ca^{2+} levels in the blood, by promoting bone resorption and increasing renal calcium resorption.

Oxyphil cells contain abundant mitochondria, do not secrete PTH, but may differentiate into chief cells.

Adrenal glands

These are a pair of glands, one associated with each kidney. Each gland contains two main regions, an outer cortex and an inner medulla, which contain different types of endocrine tissue (Fig. 40c). The embryological origin of the cortex is similar to that of the gonads. The embryological origin of the medulla is similar to that of the sympathetic nervous system.

Adrenal cortex

The cortex contains three regions (Fig. 40c) which secrete different hormones, all of which are based on cholesterol (steroid hormones).

• **Zona glomerulosa:** The zona glomerulosa (ZG) is the outermost zone of the adrenal cortex. It secretes **mineralocorticoids**, which are important for fluid homeostasis (e.g., aldosterone, which regulates absorption/uptake of K^+ and Na^+ levels in the kidney). The secretory cells are arranged in irregular ovoid clusters (glomeruli) surrounded by trabeculae, which contain capillaries. The nuclei of the cells stain strongly, and the cytoplasm of these cells is darker than those in the next zone, the zona fasciculata, as there are fewer lipid droplets in these cells.

• **Zona fasciculata:** The zona fasciculata (ZF) is the middle zone of the adrenal cortex. It secretes **glucocorticoids**, which are important for carbohydrate, protein, and lipid metabolism (e.g., cortisol, which raises blood glucose and cellular synthesis of glycogen). The pituitary hormone **adrenocorticotropic hormone** (ACTH) regulates cortisol secretion. The secretory cells are arranged in cords, often one cell thick, surrounded by fine strands of supporting tissue. The nuclei stain strongly, the cytoplasm looks pale and 'foamy' due to the lipid droplets, and it is rich in smooth endoplasmic reticulum (ER) and mitochondria.

• **Zona reticularis:** The zona reticularis (ZR) is the innermost layer of the cortex. It secretes **sex hormones** (androgens) and small amounts of **glucocorticoids**.

Adrenal medulla

This region contains strongly basophilic staining cells (they do not contain any lipid in their cytoplasm; Fig. 40c).

These cells actively secrete peptide-based hormones, for example, the catecholamines **norepinephrine (noradrenaline)** and **epinephrine (adrenaline)**.

This region is rich in venous channels, which drain blood from the sinusoids of the cortex, pass through the medulla, and drain into the medullary vein.

The sympathetic nervous system controls secretion of these hormones. Their targets are the adrenergic receptors in the heart, blood vessels, bronchioles, visceral muscle, skeletal muscle, and in the liver, where they promote glycolysis (breakdown of glycogen).

Pituitary and pineal glands, and the endocrine pancreas

41

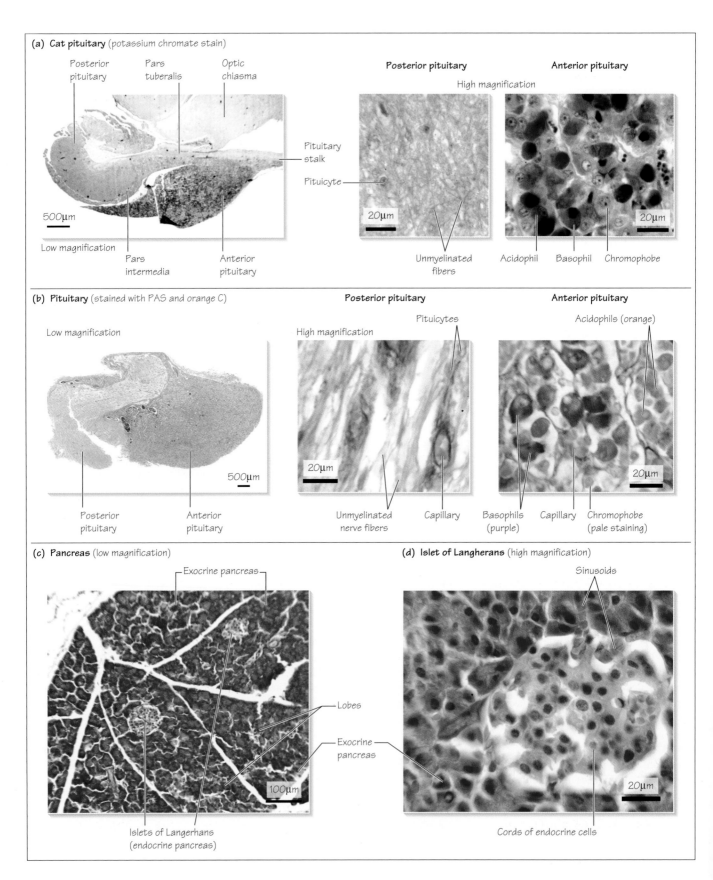

(a) Cat pituitary (potassium chromate stain)

Posterior pituitary
Pars tuberalis
Optic chiasma

Pituitary stalk

Pituicyte

500μm

Low magnification

Pars intermedia
Anterior pituitary

Posterior pituitary

High magnification

20μm

Unmyelinated fibers

Anterior pituitary

Acidophil   Basophil   Chromophobe

20μm

(b) Pituitary (stained with PAS and orange C)

Low magnification

500μm

Posterior pituitary
Anterior pituitary

Posterior pituitary

Pituicytes

High magnification

20μm

Unmyelinated nerve fibers   Capillary

Anterior pituitary

Acidophils (orange)

20μm

Basophils (purple)   Capillary   Chromophobe (pale staining)

(c) Pancreas (low magnification)

Exocrine pancreas

Lobes

Exocrine pancreas

100μm

Islets of Langerhans (endocrine pancreas)

(d) Islet of Langherans (high magnification)

Sinusoids

20μm

Cords of endocrine cells

The pituitary gland

The pituitary (or 'hypophysis') is found at the base of the brain, is about 1 cm in diameter, and has two functional regions, the anterior and posterior lobes (Fig. 41a,b).

The histological structure of the anterior and posterior lobes is different, and this reflects their different embryological origins.
• The **posterior region (neurohypophysis)** originates from nervous tissue in the brain – a downgrowth of the diencephalon).
• The **anterior region (adenohypophysis)** originates from oral ectoderm, a primitive oral cavity called **Rathke's pouch**, the remnants of which can still be seen in sections. This region is the glandular epithelial part of the pituitary, and it includes the anterior pituitary, pars intermedia, and pars tuberalis.

The **pars intermedia** (poorly developed in humans) is found in a narrow region in the posterior part of the anterior pituitary and it also has its embryological origin in Rathke's pouch.

The anterior pituitary gland

This region contains cords of epithelial cells, surrounded by a small amount of supporting connective tissue, and fenestrated capillaries (Fig. 41a,b). These cells secrete hormone in response to signals from the hypothalamus.

There are **three types** of endocrine cell:
1 **acidophils**, which stain strongly with acidic dyes;
2 **basophils**, which stain strongly with basic dyes, and stain strongly with periodic acid–Schiff due to their high glycoprotein content;
3 **chromophobes** (weakly staining), which are resting (degranulated) chromophils.

Acidophils and **basophils** secrete five different types of hormone, which are secreted into the surrounding fenestrated capillaries.

Acidophils are made up of two main types of cell, which each secrete one type of peptide hormone, as follows.
• **Somatotrophs** (40–50% of cells) secrete the growth hormone (somatotropin), the main target of which is the chondrocytes in epithelial growth plates.
• **Mammotrophs** (~15%) secrete prolactin that stimulates milk-producing tissue in the breast.

Basophils are made up of three main types of cell, which secrete glycoprotein hormones, as follows.
• **Corticotrophs** (~20%) secrete adrenocorticotropic hormone (ACTH), which targets the adrenal gland.
• **Thyrotrophs** (~5%) secrete thyroid-stimulating hormone (TSH), which targets the thyroid gland.
• **Gonadotrophs** (~10%) secrete gonadotropins. These include **follicle-stimulating hormone** (FSH), which targets the follicular cells of the ovaries (in women) or Sertoli cells of the testis (in men) and **luteinizing hormone** (LH), which promotes ovulation in women, or stimulates androgen release from the Leydig cells of testes in men.

The different subtypes of acidophils and basophils cannot be distinguished by H&E or other histological stains, but can be distinguished by immunohistochemical techniques.

The posterior pituitary gland

The posterior pituitary looks very different to the anterior pituitary (Fig. 41a,b). It contains non-myelinated axons, (neurosecretory cells), the cell bodies of which are located in the hypothalamus, together with supporting glial cells (**pituicytes**), which are similar to astrocytes, and fenestrated capillaries.

The posterior pituitary only secretes two hormones.
• **Antidiuretic hormone** (ADH) acts on the kidney to regulate water excretion, and can also act as a vasoconstrictor. Its secretion is triggered by an increase in osmotic pressure in the blood.
• **Oxytocin** acts on the uterus, causing the smooth muscle to contract during labor, and on myoepithelial cells in the mammary gland to cause milk secretion.

The pineal gland

The pineal gland is a small gland, 6–8 mm long, found close to the hypothalamus in the brain (not shown here). It secretes the hormone melatonin, which regulates the circadian rhythms of the body. Secretions of this hormone at night cause a hypnotic effect.

The endocrine pancreas

The endocrine part of the pancreas (Fig. 41c) consists of isolated islands of lighter-staining cells called islets of Langerhans (about 2% of the total volume).

Islets of Langerhans contain cords of endocrine secretory cells (up to around 3000), surrounded by fenestrated capillaries, and supported by reticulin fibers, in a delicate capsule around each islet (Fig. 41d).

The islets are **paler** than the surrounding exocrine cells, as the cells have less rough endoplasmic reticulum (ER). They contain three types of secretory cells, which cannot be distinguished by H&E staining, as follows.
• **Alpha cells** (~20%), which are peripherally located. These cells secrete glucagon, in response to lowered levels of blood glucose. Glucagon acts on the liver to raise glucose levels.
• **Beta cells** (70%), which are centrally located. These cells secrete insulin in response to increased levels of blood glucose. Insulin acts on the liver, striated muscle, fibroblasts, and adipocytes to increase glucose uptake.
  • Loss or damage to beta cells in children causes type 1 diabetes mellitus (insulin-dependent diabetes mellitus), and a consequent lifelong dependence on exogenous insulin. Type 2 diabetes mellitus (non-insulin-dependent) normally has a later onset, is commonly linked to obesity, and is caused by insulin resistance (reduced responsiveness to insulin), and the inability of the beta cells to increase insulin production.
  • **Delta cells** (~10%), which are peripherally located. These cells secrete gastrin and somatostatin. Somatostatin appears to inhibit insulin and glucagon secretion.

Each islet is supplied by up to three arterioles, which form the branching network of fenestrated capillaries, into which the hormones are secreted.

Each islet is drained by about six venules, which pass between the exocrine acini to the interlobular veins.

42 Thymus and lymph nodes

(a) The thymus (primary lymphoid tissue)

Septa (trabeculae) Lobules Cortex

Blood vessels

Medulla

1000μm

(b) Cortex (high magnification)

Developing thymocytes (developing T-lymphocytes)

Capillary

Cortical epithelioreticular cells (ectodermic origin)

20μm

(c) Medulla (high magnification)

Hassall's corpuscle containing keratinized epithelioreticular cells

Medullary epithelial cell (endodermal origin)

20μm

(d) Diagram of the lymph node

Cortex Lymphatic nodule

Follicle

High endothelial venule

Subcapsular sinus

Afferent lymphatic vessels

Medulla

Vein Efferent lymph vessel

Artery

Hilum

Capsule

Trabeculae

The medulla contains medullary cords and sinuses (not shown in diagram). Afferent lymph drains into cortical sinuses, through into medullary sinuses before leaving via efferent lymph vessels

(e) The lymph node (low magnification)

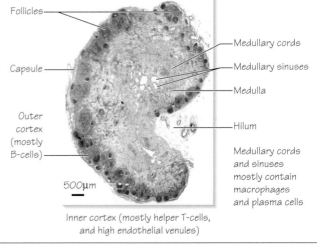

Follicles

Medullary cords

Capsule

Medullary sinuses

Medulla

Outer cortex (mostly B-cells)

Hilum

Medullary cords and sinuses mostly contain macrophages and plasma cells

500μm

Inner cortex (mostly helper T-cells, and high endothelial venules)

(f) High endothelial venule in inner cortex

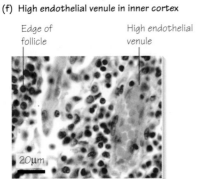

Edge of follicle

High endothelial venule

20μm

(g) Follicles in the outer cortex

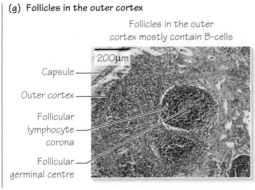

Follicles in the outer cortex mostly contain B-cells

Capsule

Outer cortex

Follicular lymphocyte corona

Follicular germinal centre

200μm

(h) Network of cells in the outer cortex

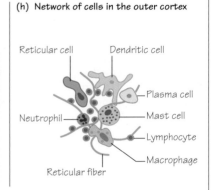

Reticular cell Dendritic cell

Plasma cell

Neutrophil Mast cell

Lymphocyte

Macrophage

Reticular fiber

The lymphatic system includes all of the various tissues that are important in mounting an immune response, including the lymphatic vessels.

It also includes all the cells involved in the immune response: lymphocytes and supporting cells (reticular cells, macrophages, dendritic cells, Langerhans cells, and epithelioreticular cells). These different cells are analysed clinically using specific 'cluster of differentiation markers' (CD), antigens expressed on the cell surface, characteristic of cell type and differentiation state.

The bone marrow and the thymus are **primary lymphatic organs**. T- and B-lymphocytes are both born in the bone marrow (Chapter 14), but T-lymphocytes need to be matured in the thymus.

Encapsulated lymphoid tissues (spleen, tonsils, and lymph nodes) are all **secondary lymphatic organs** (sites where lymphocytes respond to antigens and differentiate).

Lymphoid tissues can have efferent or both afferent and efferent lymphatic vessels. Lymphatic vessels are networks of 'blind' capillaries found in loose connective tissue. They are most common in the dermis of skin and in mucous membranes (e.g., in the gut (see Chapter 26), respiratory system (Chapter 31) and oral cavities). The fluid in lymph is derived from the fluid and substances that filter out of capillaries, and from interstitial (extracellular) spaces. The lymph vessels also transport dietary lipids. The lymph eventually drains into venous blood. Lymphocytes travel in the blood and in the lymph.

Primary lymphatic organ
Thymus gland
This is a primary lymphoid tissue. It is active in children but starts to atrophy at puberty.

The thymus gland responsible for the
- maturation of immunocompetent T-lymphocytes;
- proliferation of mature T-cell clones;
- developing immunological self-tolerance;
- secretion of hormones for T-cell growth and development.

The thymus contains two lobes divided up into lobules by septa, and is covered by an outer connective tissue capsule (Fig. 42a). It does not have afferent lymphatics, but does have efferent lymphatics. All cells (including white blood cells) entering the thymus do so from the blood.

The **cortex** (Fig. 42b) is the outer, more darkly (basophilic) staining region, and it contains more lymphocytes than the inner lighter staining region (the **medulla**).

T-cell progenitors proliferate and develop in the cortex. Only 5% of the T-cell clones, which recognize self-MHC encoded surface glycoproteins, and therefore will be self-immunotolerant, survive.

Differentiating T-lymphocytes (thymocytes) associate with the reticular epithelial (epithelioreticular) cells (Fig. 42b). Survivors either leave the thymus via venules and efferent lymphatics along the border between the cortex and the medulla, or they pass into the medulla, where they are further selected by thymic dendritic cells and matured before passing out of the medullary venules and efferent lymphatics.

Cortical epithelial cells have a reticular (net-like) organization. They form tightly connected sheaths around capillaries entering the thymus, blocking the entry of antigenic material into the spaces between them (the **blood–thymus barrier**).

In addition, cortical epithelial cells secrete the hormones for T-cell growth and development (thymosin, thymulin, and thymopoietin).

The medulla (Fig. 42c) contains **Hassall's corpuscles**, which contain flat, non-secreting, keratinized epithelial cells (type VI epithelioreticular cells), arranged in concentric layers. They secrete cytokines and thymic stromal lymphopoietin, which activates dendritic cells.

Secondary lymphatic organs
Lymph nodes
The lymph nodes include about 100–200 bean-shaped lymph nodes along lymphatic vessels in the neck, thorax, abdomen, and pelvis. They contain B- and T-lymphocytes (most of which enter via the bloodstream), and macrophages. They monitor the content of blood and lymph for foreign antigenic material.

A **capsule** of dense connective tissue covers the lymph nodes (Fig. 42d,e). Extensions of this tissue called **trabeculae** provide support for blood vessels.

Lymph nodes are divided up into a cortex and a medulla, and the **cortex** is further divided into an **outer** and **inner** (or deep) cortex (Fig. 42e).

Lymph, containing micro-organisms, soluble antigens, antigen-presenting cells, and some B-cells, enters through **afferent lymphatic** vessels in the **subcapsular sinus**. However, most B- and T-lymphocytes enter the lymph nodes through specialized venules, found in the inner cortex. These are called **high endothelial venules** and are lined by a discontinuous layer of simple squamous endothelium (Fig. 42f). (They are also found in Peyer's patches and the thymus.)

Lymph runs through **sinuses** in the cortex into **sinuses** in the medulla and leaves in **efferent lymphatic vessels** at the **hilum**. **Efferent lymph** contains T-lymphocytes, B-cells, plasma cells, and antibodies.

Lymph node cortex
Primary nodules/follicles in the **outer cortex** (Fig. 42g) mostly contain B-lymphocytes (B-cells). They sit in the spaces between reticular fibers. When activated by T-cells, B-cells proliferate, forming antibody-secreting **plasma** cells and these **secondary nodules** develop a central, lighter-staining area (**germinal centre**). Plasma cells live for ~3 days, and secrete IgG type antibodies.

The outer cortex also contains **macrophages, dendritic cells**, and some **T-lymphocytes**. Macrophages and dendritic cells trap antigens and present them to B-lymphocytes (Fig. 42h).

The **inner cortex** does not contain nodules, but does contain the majority of T-cells (helper T-lymphocytes). The **medullary lymphatic sinuses** contain reticular cells and macrophages, which sample the lymph.

In the **medulla**, the medullary cords and sinuses contain plasma cells, macrophages and B-cells. Activated B-cells secrete antibodies directly into the medullary sinuses.

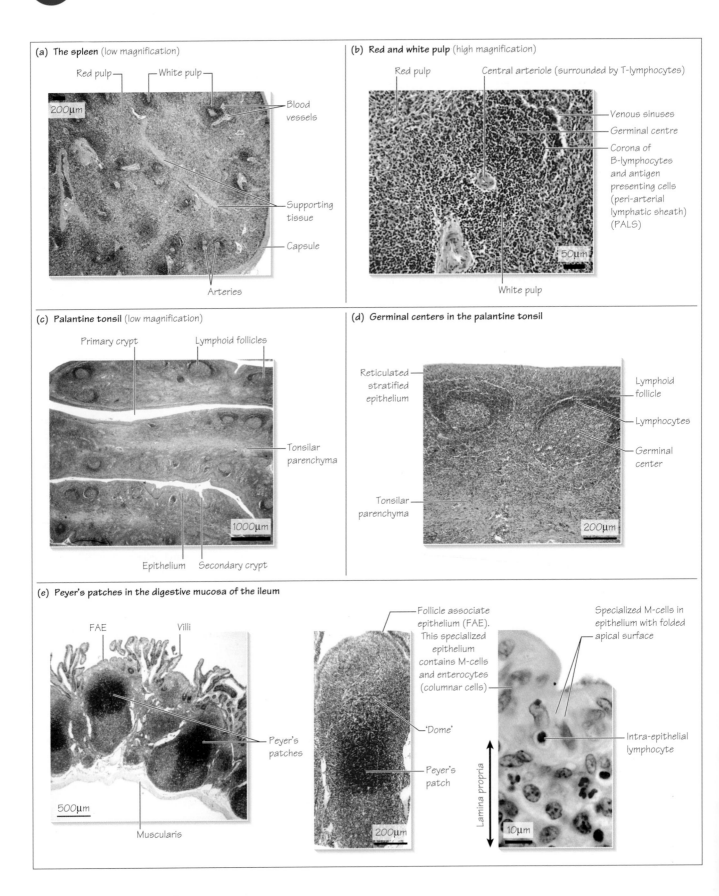

(a) The spleen (low magnification)

Red pulp — White pulp —

200μm

Blood vessels

Supporting tissue

Capsule

Arteries

(b) Red and white pulp (high magnification)

Red pulp — Central arteriole (surrounded by T-lymphocytes)

Venous sinuses

Germinal centre

Corona of B-lymphocytes and antigen presenting cells (peri-arterial lymphatic sheath) (PALS)

50μm

White pulp

(c) Palantine tonsil (low magnification)

Primary crypt — Lymphoid follicles

Tonsilar parenchyma

1000μm

Epithelium — Secondary crypt

(d) Germinal centers in the palantine tonsil

Reticulated stratified epithelium

Lymphoid follicle

Lymphocytes

Germinal center

Tonsilar parenchyma

200μm

(e) Peyer's patches in the digestive mucosa of the ileum

FAE — Villi

Peyer's patches

500μm

Muscularis

Follicle associate epithelium (FAE). This specialized epithelium contains M-cells and enterocytes (columnar cells)

'Dome'

Peyer's patch

200μm

Lamina propria

Specialized M-cells in epithelium with folded apical surface

Intra-epithelial lymphocyte

10μm

Spleen

The spleen is a secondary encapsulated lymphoid organ, found between the stomach and the diaphragm. It is important for:
1 antibody production;
2 facilitating immune responses to blood-borne antigens;
3 eliminating worn-out blood cells and platelets.

The spleen is the largest mass of lymphatic tissue in the body, and is also the body's largest blood filter.

A dense capsule covers the spleen (Fig. 43a), and connective tissue trabeculae emanate from this capsule to provide support for the blood vessels entering the spleen. There are efferent but no afferent lymphatics.

The spleen contains two main regions, related to their function: **red** and **white pulp**.

Red pulp

This region (Fig. 43b) removes old erythrocytes from the circulation and recycles iron from these cells.
• The afferent splenic artery enters the spleen via the hilum, and branches into arterioles in areas of white pulp.
• These arterioles end in cords in the red pulp.
• The cords contain fibroblasts and reticular fibers but the blood vessels do not have an endothelial lining.
• The blood leaves the cords by entering adjacent venous sinuses. These are lined by a discontinuous epithelium.
• This arrangement means that blood cells are forced through slits between the cells in the cords in order to enter the venous sinuses.
• Older erythrocytes become stuck in the cords because they have stiffer membranes and cannot move through the slits.
• These cells are phagocytosed by macrophages in the red pulp, and their iron is recycled and stored as ferritin.

White pulp

This region (Fig. 43b) contains lymphoid aggregations, in which B- and T-lymphocytes are separated into different compartments, arranged around branching arterioles.

T-lymphocytes are found in the **periarteriolar lymphoid sheath** (PALS) where they interact with dendritic cells and B-lymphocytes.

B-lymphocytes are found in **follicles**.

The **marginal zone**, which lies between red and white pulp, is an important transit area in which lymphoid cells leave the blood and enter the white pulp. Specialized macrophages in this region are involved in the innate immune response.

B-lymphocytes in this region rapidly differentiate into IgM-secreting plasma cells in response to blood-borne pathogens. Alternatively, they can become antigen-presenting cells, enter the white pulp, and elicit an immune response as part of the adaptive immune reaction.

Tonsils

Tonsils are secondary partially encapsulated masses of lymphoid tissue (Fig. 43c). There is a ring of tonsilar tissue in the pharynx, which includes adenoids (the nasopharyngeal tonsils), paired tubal tonsils, the lingual tonsil, and palatine tonsils (Fig. 43c).

A stratified squamous epithelium covers the outer (**luminal**) surface in common with the oral mucosa.

In humans, the tonsils contain many invaginations that form **blind crypts**, whose surface is covered by a modified (reticulated) stratified epithelium.

Here, specialized epithelial cells (similar to M-cells in Peyer's patches, see below) phagocytose bacterial antigens, and then secrete them into the interstitial spaces, where they are endocytosed by lymphoid cells.

The epithelium also contains T-lymphocytes and activated B-lymphocytes, which secrete antibodies.

The lymphoid follicles, lying below the epithelium, contain most of the immunocompetent cells.

These contain germinal centers similar to those found in lymph nodes (Fig. 43d). Activated cells mostly secrete IgA-type antibodies.

The tonsils do not filter lymph.

Peyer's patches and lymphoid aggregations

Peyer's patches are non-encapsulated lymphoid aggregations, that respond to antigens close to wet mucosal surface. They are also known as mucosa-associated lymphoid tissue or MALT (or gut-associated lymphoid tissue; GALT). Other lymphoid aggregations are found around the body, for example in the lungs (see Chapter 31).

Peyer's patches (Fig. 43e) play an important role in sampling foreign antigens in the digestive tract, distinguishing commensal from foreign bacteria.

The epithelium lying above the Peyer's patch (Fig. 43e) contains specialized flat epithelial cells called M- (membrane or microfold) cells or FAE (follicle-associated epithelial) cells. This region of the epithelium does not contain goblet cells or subepithelial myofibroblasts.

The M-cells do not have highly organized microvilli (Fig. 43e) or secrete digestive enzymes, but they do have small microfolds on their apical surfaces. M-cells form pockets towards their basal surface, which enclose lymphocytes. Dendritic cells lie close to the M-cells, and extend processes across the tight junctions between the epithelial cells.

Antigens taken up by either M-cells or dendritic cells are transferred to lymphocytes, which then present the antigens to antigen-presenting cells underneath the epithelium. These cells then transfer or present the antigen to T-lymphocytes, which enter Peyer's patch via a postcapillary high endothelial venule (see Chapter 42).

The germinal center of Peyer's patches contains B-cells, which differentiate into Ig-A secreting plasma cells, when stimulated. These antibodies are then secreted directly onto the gut lumen, help to prevent micro-organisms in the gut from sticking to the gut epithelium, and can neutralize toxins and viruses.

The 'dome' around the germinal center contains T-cells, macrophages, and plasma cells.

Peyer's patches do not have any afferent lymphatics. Activated lymphocytes pass out in the efferent lymphatics and travel to the lymph nodes.

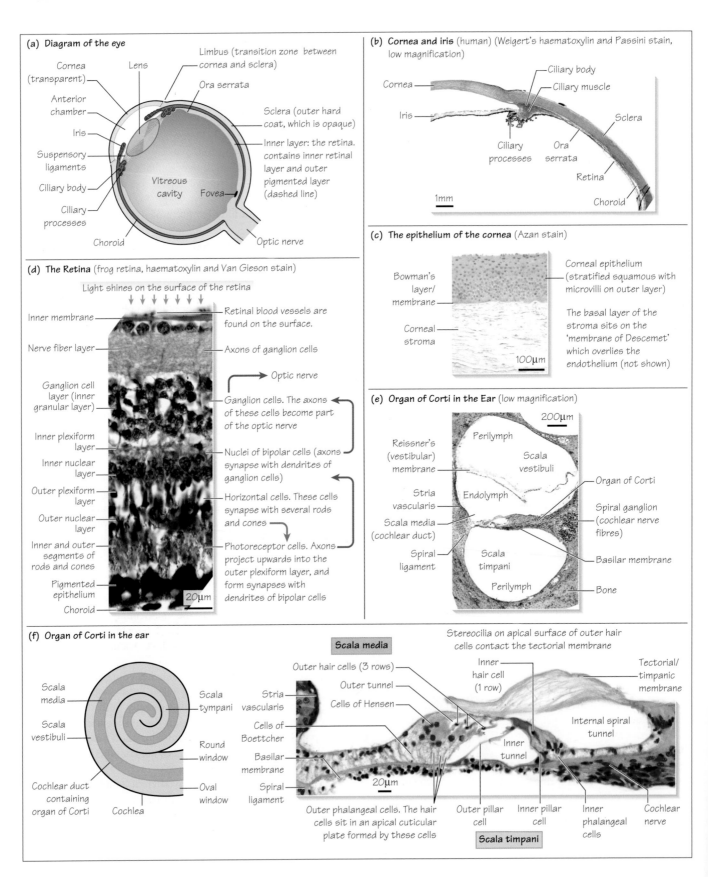

(a) Diagram of the eye

Cornea (transparent)
Lens
Limbus (transition zone between cornea and sclera)
Ora serrata
Anterior chamber
Iris
Suspensory ligaments
Ciliary body
Ciliary processes
Choroid
Vitreous cavity
Fovea
Sclera (outer hard coat, which is opaque)
Inner layer: the retina. contains inner retinal layer and outer pigmented layer (dashed line)
Optic nerve

(b) Cornea and iris (human) (Weigert's haematoxylin and Passini stain, low magnification)

Cornea
Iris
Ciliary processes
Ciliary body
Ciliary muscle
Sclera
Ora serrata
Retina
Choroid
1mm

(c) The epithelium of the cornea (Azan stain)

Bowman's layer/membrane
Corneal stroma
Corneal epithelium (stratified squamous with microvilli on outer layer)
The basal layer of the stroma sits on the 'membrane of Descemet' which overlies the endothelium (not shown)
100μm

(d) The Retina (frog retina, haematoxylin and Van Gieson stain)

Light shines on the surface of the retina

Inner membrane
Nerve fiber layer
Ganglion cell layer (inner granular layer)
Inner plexiform layer
Inner nuclear layer
Outer plexiform layer
Outer nuclear layer
Inner and outer segments of rods and cones
Pigmented epithelium
Choroid
20μm

Retinal blood vessels are found on the surface.
Axons of ganglion cells
Optic nerve
Ganglion cells. The axons of these cells become part of the optic nerve
Nuclei of bipolar cells (axons synapse with dendrites of ganglion cells)
Horizontal cells. These cells synapse with several rods and cones
Photoreceptor cells. Axons project upwards into the outer plexiform layer, and form synapses with dendrites of bipolar cells

(e) Organ of Corti in the Ear (low magnification)

200μm
Reissner's (vestibular) membrane
Stria vascularis
Scala media (cochlear duct)
Spiral ligament
Perilymph
Scala vestibuli
Endolymph
Scala timpani
Perilymph
Organ of Corti
Spiral ganglion (cochlear nerve fibres)
Basilar membrane
Bone

(f) Organ of Corti in the ear

Scala media
Scala vestibuli
Cochlear duct containing organ of Corti
Cochlea
Scala tympani
Round window
Oval window

Scala media
Stria vascularis
Cells of Boettcher
Basilar membrane
Spiral ligament
Outer hair cells (3 rows)
Outer tunnel
Cells of Hensen
Outer phalangeal cells. The hair cells sit in an apical cuticular plate formed by these cells
Stereocilia on apical surface of outer hair cells contact the tectorial membrane
Inner hair cell (1 row)
Inner tunnel
Outer pillar cell
Inner pillar cell
Scala timpani
Internal spiral tunnel
Inner phalangeal cells
Tectorial/timpanic membrane
Cochlear nerve
20μm

The eye

The eyes are sensory organs specialized for sight. The cornea and the lens capture and focus the light. The photoreceptors in the retina detect light intensity and color, and convert this information into electrical impulses, which are carried out of the eye to the brain, by the optic nerve. Each eye captures a slight different image of the same field, which are interpreted by the brain to generate a 3D image.

The eye lies in a bony socket, and six extrinsic 'extra-ocular' muscles connected to the eye control its movement. The eyeball (Fig. 44a) contains an outer fibrous layer, the **corneoscleral** coat, which includes the outer **sclera** (white, and opaque) over most of the eyeball, and the transparent **cornea** at the front of the eye (Fig. 44b).

The **sclera** contains flat collagen bundles and fibroblasts, nerves, and blood vessels. It is continuous with the **cornea** (Fig. 44b).

The **ciliary body**, found between the cornea and the sclera, contains a region of smooth muscle (ciliary muscle), which changes the shape of the **lens** (accommodation) so that it focuses light on the retina. The **lens** is suspended between the edges of the ciliary body by zonular fibers, and consists of a thick basal lamina (lens capsule), subcapsular epithelium (anterior surface), and lens fibers which form from the epithelial cells, elongating, losing their nuclei, and becoming filled with the protein crystallin. The lens is normally transparent. However, when **cataracts** form, the lens loses its transparency.

The **iris**, which lies behind the cornea and in front of the lens, is a contractile diaphragm, and its central aperture (hole) is called the **pupil**. The iris contains smooth muscle, which acts to change the size of the pupil and pigmented cells. Changing pupil size controls the amount of light that reaches the retina (adaptation). The heavily pigmented retina is visible through the pupil (aperture), and thus the pupil looks black.

The cornea

The cornea (~0.5 mm thick in the central region) contains a **stratified squamous epithelium** (Fig. 44c). Unlike the skin, this layer contains ferritin (an iron storage protein) to protect against DNA damage, instead of melanin (which would reduce the opacity of the eye). The underlying thick (10 μm) basement membrane (Bowman's membrane) helps to prevent infections.

A layer of corneal 'stroma' lies underneath the basement membrane (substantia propria). It contains about 60 thin lamellae: collagen fibrils arranged in parallel bundles, with the bundles in one layer arranged at right angles to those in the next. This arrangement gives the cornea its transparency. Corneal endothelial cells line the interior surface of the stroma, supported by a thick basal lamina (Descemet's membrane).

The sclera surrounds the middle layer of choroid (a highly pigmented vascular layer).

The retina

The retina forms the innermost layer and contains two main regions:
• an outer **non-photosensitive portion** consisting of **pigmented epithelium** (retinal pigment epithelium, RPE), which contains **simple cuboidal pigmented** cells;
• an inner **photosensitive portion** (Fig. 44d), which contains conducting neurons (bipolar and ganglion cells), associated neurons (horizontal, centrifugal, and amacrine) and supporting cells arranged into layers above the basal layer which contains the photoreceptors (rods, ~100×10^6 and cones, ~7×10^6). Rods are more sensitive to light. Cones are sensitive to different wavelengths of light.

Supporting cells (Müller's and neuroglial cells) are also present throughout these layers.

Light has to pass through the layers of conducting neurons before reaching the photoreceptors. The resulting nerve impulses are carried out via the axonal processes of the ganglion cells that lie parallel on the surface of the retina, and out through the optic nerve.

The ear

The ear contains three chambers, and is important for hearing (auditory system) and for balance (vestibular system). The structures in the ear that perform these two functions are derived from surface ectoderm in the embryo.

The **external ear** consists of the auricle or pinna, the external acoustic meatus (air-filled space, 25 mm long), ceruminous glands, and the eardrum (tympanic membrane). The elastic cartilage in the pinna holds its shape.

The middle ear (tympanic cavity), another air-filled space, contains the auditory tube (eustachian tube), three small bones (the auditory ossicles), and the muscles that move these bones. Sound waves entering the ear are converted into mechanical vibrations, with the help of the ossicles, and transmitted to the inner ear via the oval (cochlear) window. The eustachian tube connects the middle ear to the nasopharynx.

The inner ear contains the bony labyrinth, and within it, the membranous labyrinth. The membranous labyrinth contains endolymph, which is rich in K^+ and low in Na^+ ions.

The bony labyrinth is made up of **semicircular canals**, the **vestibule**, and the **cochlea**. The semicircular canals are important for balance. The cochlea (a cone-shaped helix) is important for hearing. Both of these are connected to the vestibule.

The cochlea duct is divided into **three parts (canals)**:
• two outer canals called **scala vestibuli** and **scala timpani**, both of which contain **perilymph**;
• an inner canal called the **scala media**.

Reissner's and the basilar membrane separate the scala media from the two outer canals, and the **scala media** contains **endolymph**, produced by the stria vascularis. It is richer in K^+ and lower in Na^+ than perilymph.

The spiral **organ of Corti**, an epithelial layer found on the floor of the **scala media**, senses the mechanical vibrations transmitted to the oval window by the auditory ossicles (Fig. 44e,f). It contains inner and outer hair cells, supporting cells, the tectorial membrane, an inner tunnel, which is lined by inner and outer pillar cells, and various supporting cells such as the phalangeal cells.

Mechanical vibrations traveling into the inner ear are transmitted to both the perilymph and endolymph, and a traveling wave is set up in the basilar membrane. A specific frequency of sound displaces part of the basilar membrane, and the tectorial membrane also vibrates. This generates a shearing effect between the basilar and tectorial membranes, displacing the stereocilia of the hair cells. The mechanical distortion causes channels in the outer hair cells to open, K^+ ions enter, the hair cells become depolarized, and a stimulus is produced, which is sent to the brain by the cochlear nerve.

Self-test questions

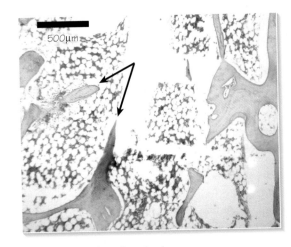

Fig. A Section through white matter of the spinal cord.

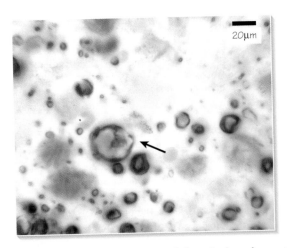

Fig. D Section through trabecular bone.

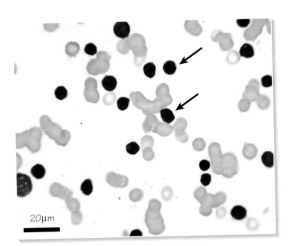

Fig. B Blood smear.

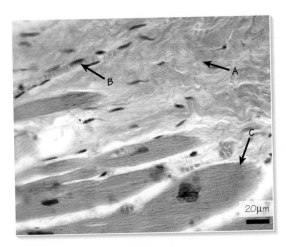

Fig. E Section through the myocardium of the heart.

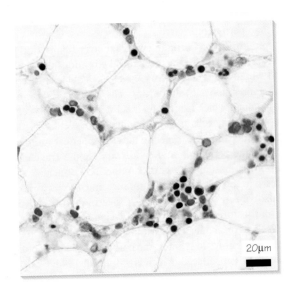

Fig. C Bone marrow smear (30-year-old).

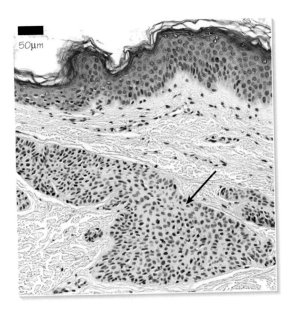

Fig. F Section through the skin.

 Histology at a Glance, 1st edition. © Michelle Peckham. Published 2011 by Blackwell Publishing Ltd.

Chapters 1–4: Introduction to histology

1 Are tissues stained before being fixed?
2 What does hematoxylin stain and why?
3 Do microscope objectives with a large numerical aperture have a lower resolution than those with a small numerical aperture?
4 PAS is used to visualize what type of substance (protein, carbohydrate or DNA)?
5 What are histological sections normally embedded in before sectioning?

Chapters 5 and 6: The cell

6 What protein are microfilaments composed of?
7 What is the function of desmosomes?
8 What is the site of ribosomal RNA production in the nucleus?
9 Which organelle produces most of the cell's energy in the form of ATP?
10 What is the difference between rough and smooth ER?

Chapter 7: Epithelium

11 What do epithelia cover?
12 Are all the cells in a stratified epithelium in contact with the basement membrane?
13 What type of specialization found on the apical surfaces of cells contains microtubules?
14 What is the function of goblet cells?
15 What types of filament are found in adherens junctions?

Chapters 8 and 9: Skeletal, cardiac, and smooth muscle

16 Is skeletal muscle voluntary or involuntary?
17 Does smooth muscle contain cross-striations?
18 What types of cell junction are found in intercalated discs?
19 Which organelle acts as the intracellular store for Ca^{2+} in skeletal muscle?
20 Which type of muscle is multinucleated?

Chapters 10 and 11: Nerves and supporting cells in the CNS and PNS

21 Which structure between neurons conducts the nerve impulse between one neuron and the next?
22 How do microglial cells respond to tissue damage?
23 Does the CNS contain aggregates of cell bodies called ganglia?
24 Where are the cell bodies for motor neurons found?
25 Write a short report on the image shown in Fig. A, which is a section through white matter in the spinal cord. What is the arrow (A) pointing to?

Chapter 12: Connective tissue

26 What type of connective tissue is found in tendons?
27 What are glycosoaminoglycans (GAGs), and what did GAGs used to be called?

28 Which types of immune cell in connective tissue produce histamine?
29 Which types of fiber are found in connective tissue?

Chapters 13 and 14: Blood and hemopoiesis

30 What important organelle do erythrocytes not contain?
31 Which bones contain hemopoietic marrow?
32 Precursor blood cells contain nuclei with non-condensed chromatin and a cytoplasm rich in free ribosomes; what does this tell you about their activity?
33 What type of cell generates platelets?
34 In the image shown in Fig. B of a blood smear, what are the arrows pointing to? Is there anything unusual about this blood smear, and if so, what is it?
35 In the image shown in Fig. C, of the bone marrow from a 30-year-old, does the bone marrow look normal?

Chapters 15 and 16: Bone and cartilage

36 Which cells secrete the matrix of cartilage?
37 What type of GAG does hyaline cartilage contain?
38 What type of fiber does hyaline cartilage contain?
39 Why is bone harder than cartilage?
40 What would a pathologist conclude about the image shown in Fig. D, and what are the arrows pointing to?

Chapters 17–19: Cardiovascular system

41 Why do the walls of the cardiovascular system have a single layer of muscle while those of the gastrointestinal tract have two or sometimes three layers of muscle?
42 How do Purkinje cells differ from normal cardiac muscle cells?
43 What is the predominant layer in elastic arteries and what does it contain?
44 What are the small blood vessels in the tunica adventitia of the aorta called, and what is their function?
45 How does the structure of the tunica media in a muscular artery differ from that of an elastic artery?
46 In what direction do the muscle fibers in the tunica media of muscular arteries run? What is the significance of this?
47 What are fenestrated capillaries?
48 What are the arrows (A), (B), and (C) pointing to in the image of the myocardium shown in Fig. E? What would a pathologist conclude from this image?

Chapters 20–22: Skin

49 How does the epidermis of thick skin differ from thin skin?
50 In which layer of the epidermis does mitosis occur?
51 Which cells synthesize melanin?
52 What does dendritic mean?
53 What is hair made of?
54 What is the small invagination of dermal tissue at the base of hairs called, and what does it contain?
55 Does the nail bed contribute to nail growth?
56 What are the large empty cells called in the hypodermis of skin?
57 What would a pathologist conclude from the image of the skin shown in Fig. F, and what is the arrow pointing to?

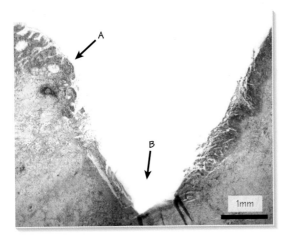

Fig. G Section through the stomach.

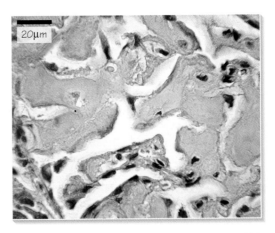

Fig. J Section through part of the glomerulus in the kidney (high magnification).

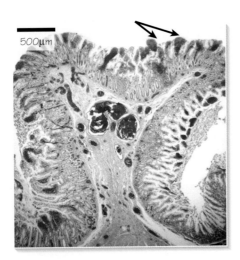

Fig. H Section through the colon.

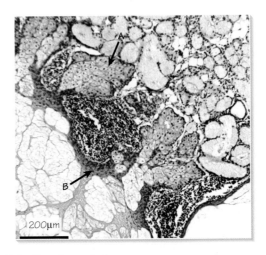

Fig. K Section through the ovary.

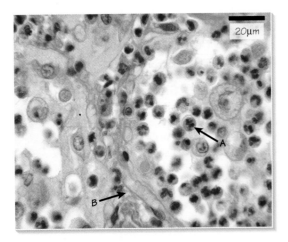

Fig. I Section through the lung.

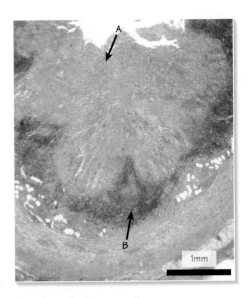

Fig. L Section through the appendix.

Chapters 23–28: Digestive system

58 Why is the vermilion border red (in living people)?

59 What is the function of the papillae on the tongue?

60 Which type of papilla is keratinized?

61 Acini are secretory units of glands; how do mucous acini differ from serous acini?

62 What are serous demilunes?

63 What happens to the saliva within striated ducts?

64 In the gut, which layer varies the most between different parts of the gastrointestinal tract?

65 How could you tell if your sections have been cut parallel or perpendicular to the long axis of the oesophagus?

66 What do the arrows in Fig. G (A) and (B) point to, and what would a pathologist conclude from this image?

67 What type of secretory cells predominates in the pyloric region?

68 What do G-cells secrete?

69 What is present in the striated (brush) border of enterocytes?

70 What do Brunner's glands secrete?

71 Do the absorptive cells of the large intestine have a striated border?

72 What is the muscle arrangement in the large intestine known as?

73 In the section through the colon shown in Fig. H, what are the arrows pointing to? Would a pathologist consider these features normal? If not, why not?

Chapter 29: Liver

(See also Chapters 28 and 41 for gall bladder and pancreas)

74 What three structures are found in the portal tract?

75 In which direction does blood run in the sinusoids?

76 What type of epithelium lines the gall bladder?

77 What stimulates the gall bladder to empty?

78 What do the acini of the pancreas synthesize?

79 What three types of secretory cells are present in the islets of Langerhans?

80 How do these secretions leave the islets, and which components of the islets facilitate this?

Chapters 30 and 31: Respiratory system

81 What are the three main types of cell found in the epithelium lining the trachea?

82 What type of cartilage is present in the walls of the trachea?

83 What is surfactant, where is it found, and which cells make it?

84 What is the approximate thickness of the interalveolar wall?

85 What are the arrows pointing towards in Fig. I, and what would a pathologist conclude about this image?

Chapters 32–34: Urinary system

86 Which region of the kidney contains renal corpuscles?

87 What is the role of the macula densa?

88 What type of epithelium lines proximal tubules?

89 What type of epithelium lines the bladder?

90 In the image shown in Fig. J, what would a pathologist make of the appearance of this glomerulus from the kidney?

Chapters 35 and 36: Female reproductive system

91 What are the major functions of the ovary?

92 What type of tissue is the theca folliculi?

93 Which cells develop into the zonula granulosa?

94 What can you conclude about the image shown of the ovary in Fig. K? What are arrows (A) and (B) pointing towards?

95 How would you expect the ovary of a prepubescent girl to look different to that of a pregnant woman?

96 What do endometrial glands secrete?

97 It is common to find accumulations of lymphoid tissue in the walls of the vagina; why do you think this is?

98 What is colostrum and where is it found?

Chapters 37–39: Male reproductive system

99 What specialized type of cell division takes place during gametogenesis, and what is its purpose?

100 What are the components of the male genital duct system?

101 What are the accessory sex glands in the male reproductive system?

102 By what route do the spermatozoa leave the seminiferous tubules?

103 What do Leydig cells secrete?

104 What type of epithelium lines the epididymis?

105 Are accessory sex glands endocrine or exocrine glands?

Chapters 40 and 41: Endocrine glands

106 From which type of tissue are glands formed?

107 What do endocrine glands secrete?

108 How is colloid converted into active thyroid hormone?

109 Cells from the zona fasciculata contain many triglyceride droplets, why is this?

Chapters 42 and 43: Lymphatic system

110 What are lymphoid aggregations in the submucosa of the small intestine called?

111 What type of lymphoid tissue are tonsils?

112 Efferent lymph drains out from lymph nodes at which structure?

113 Where are T-cells matured?

114 What would a pathologist conclude about the image shown in Fig. L?

Chapter 44: Eye and ear

115 What does the ciliary body in the eye contain?

116 What type of epithelium is on the outer surface of the cornea?

117 What type of neuron is found in the inner granular layer of the retina?

118 In which part of the eye do cataracts form?

119 What type of fluid does the scala vestibuli in the inner ear contain?

120 What is the role of the phalangeal cells?

Self-test answers

Chapters 1–4: Introduction to histology

1 No, tissues are normally fixed first, and then stained.
2 Hematoxylin stain is a basic stain that binds to acidic structures (DNA, RNA), and therefore stains the nucleus, and ribosomes.
3 No, microscope objectives with a large numerical aperture have higher resolving power.
4 PAS is used to visualize carbohydrate.
5 Histological sections are normally embedded in wax before sectioning.

Chapters 5 and 6: The cell

6 Microfilaments are composed of actin.
7 Desmosomes connect cells to each other, for example in epithelia.
8 Ribosomal RNA is made in the nucleolus.
9 Mitochondria produce most of the cell's ATP.
10 Rough ER contains ribosomes but smooth ER does not.

Chapter 7: Epithelium

11 Epithelia cover the outer surfaces of the body.
12 No, not all the cells in a stratified epithelium are in contact with the basement membrane.
13 Microtubules are found in cilia.
14 Goblet cells secrete mucus.
15 Actin filaments.

Chapters 8 and 9: Skeletal, cardiac, and smooth muscle

16 Skeletal muscle is voluntary.
17 Smooth muscle does not contain cross-striations, because the contractile filaments do not have a regular sarcomeric arrangement.
18 Intercalated discs contain adherens junctions, gap junctions, and desmosomes.
19 The sarcoplasmic reticulum is the main Ca^{2+} store in skeletal muscle.
20 Skeletal muscle is multinucleated.

Chapters 10 and 11: Nerves and supporting cells in the CNS and PNS

21 The synapse.
22 They differentiate into macrophages and engulf dead tissue.
23 No. Ganglia are found just outside the CNS.
24 The cell bodies for motor neurons are found in the spinal cord.
25 White matter is full of myelinated axons in normal tissue. In the image shown in Fig. A, there are only a few. The arrow (A) is pointing to one of these. The image is taken from a person suffering from hemiplegia, in which many neurons have died, and there will be severe muscle weakness on one side of the body.

Chapter 12: Connective tissue

26 Tendons contain dense regular connective tissue.

27 Glycosoaminoglycans are made up of a protein core bound to repeating disaccharide units. They used to be called 'ground substance'.
28 Mast cells produce histamine.
29 Fibers include collagen and elastin.

Chapters 13 and 14: Blood and hemopoiesis

30 They do not contain nuclei.
31 Hemopoietic marrow is found in the intratrabecular spaces of all bone.
32 Precursor blood cells are highly active in transcription, translation, and protein synthesis.
33 Megakaryocytes generate platelets.
34 The arrows in Fig. B are pointing to B-lymphocytes. There are more of these cells than would be expected in a normal smear. This indicates that the patient could be suffering from chronic lymphocytic leukemia. Immunocytochemistry could be used to test this diagnosis further, using antibodies for cluster of differentiation (CD) antigens as the B-lymphocytes in this type of leukemia have a characteristic pattern of CD markers on their surface.
35 Considering the age of the patient, the bone marrow smear (Fig. C) has far fewer cells than expected. There are some precursor erythroid cells, but very few precursor myeloid cells. This could be an example of aplastic anemia.

Chapters 15 and 16: Bone and cartilage

36 Chondroblasts secrete the matrix, and continue to do so as they become embedded in the matrix as chondrocytes.
37 They contain aggrecan (chondroitin sulfate bound to hyaluronic acid).
38 Hyaline cartilage contains type II collagen fibers.
39 This is because the extracellular matrix is heavily calcified.
40 In this image of trabecular bone (Fig. D), trabeculae (arrowed) look thin and the bone marrow is quite fatty, suggesting it is from an older person. The thin trabeculae suggest a bone disorder, most likely to be related to fragile bones (osteoporosis).

Chapters 17–19: Cardiovascular system

41 The layer of muscle in the cardiovascular system is circular, and can contract and relax to push blood around the body. In the gastrointestinal tract, muscle layers are both circular and longitudinal (and sometimes oblique) for peristalsis (contraction above, and relaxation below the bolus of food), to squeeze food to move it along the tract, and to help break the food down by mixing.
42 They have reduced myofibrils, do not contain intercalated discs, are larger, and do not have T-tubules.
43 The predominant layer is the tunica media layer, which contains concentric layers of elastin.
44 These are called vasa vasorum, and provide the blood supply for these larger arteries.

45 The tunica media in a muscular artery contains large amounts of smooth muscle, whereas that in an elastic artery contains large amounts of elastin.

46 They run in a circular direction, and can constrict the diameter of the vessel when they contract due to this arrangement.

47 Fenestrated capillaries contain small pores (fenestrations) to facilitate exchange between the blood and the surrounding tissue.

48 In Fig. E, the arrow (A) is pointing to connective tissue, (B) to a capillary, and (C) to a cardiomyocyte. The presence of a large amount of connective tissue in the myocardium is unusual. It looks as though the heart muscle has been damaged, and that connective tissue has replaced dead cardiomyocytes. This type of fibrosis can occur due to hypertension. Fibrosis also occurs with ageing.

Chapters 20–22: Skin

49 Thick skin has a much thicker layer of keratin, and the dermal papillae are more pronounced. Some histologists can identify an extra layer (stratum lucidum) in the epidermis.

50 Mitosis occurs in the basal layer.

51 Melanocytes synthesize melanin.

52 Dendritic means to have branching projections.

53 Hair is made of keratin (dead keratinized cells).

54 This invagination is called the dermal papilla and it contains the blood and nerve supply for the hair.

55 No, the nail bed does not contribute to nail growth.

56 These are adipocytes.

57 The arrow (Fig. F) is pointing to a large cluster of cells in the dermis that are not normally found here. The dermis mainly contains connective tissue, nerve, blood vessels, and sweat glands. In hairy skin, it also contains hairs and sebaceous glands. The cluster of cells look like melanocytes, which should be restricted to the epidermal layer. This suggests that this could be a type of skin cancer called melanoma, a malignant tumor of melanocytes.

Chapters 23–28: Digestive system

58 Because it is highly vascularized.

59 They produce a rough surface to help move food around. Some papillae also contain taste buds.

60 Filiform papillae.

61 Mucous acini secrete a more viscid (less watery) secretion that stains less strongly in sections.

62 These are serous acini that surround mucous acini, forming a seromucous acinus.

63 Striated ducts (which look striated because they have vertically aligned mitochondria in the basal membrane) are involved in resorption of water, secretion of bicarbonate, and resorption of sodium and chloride ions.

64 The mucosa layer is the layer that changes most.

65 The inner layer of muscle is circular. This would look different if it is cut in cross-section, compared to if it was cut longitudinally, and so this would tell you in which direction the section had been cut.

66 The mucosa in the regions arrowed (Fig. G) is different. It looks normal at (A) and abnormal at (B). This looks like the mucosa has become degraded. This could be a peptic ulcer, commonly caused by the bacterium *Helicobacter pylori*.

67 Mucous-secreting cells.

68 Gastrin.

69 These contain microvilli.

70 An alkaline mucus.

71 No, these cells only have very short apical microvilli.

72 It is called the taenia coli.

73 The arrows (Fig. H) are pointing toward the epithelium of the colon, which seems to be rich in blood hemorrhages. These are not normally present in the colon, and they could be a sign of chronic ulcerative colitis.

Chapter 29: Liver

74 Hepatic artery, hepatic portal vein, and bile duct.

75 From the portal tracts into the center of the lobule.

76 Tall columnar epithelium.

77 The release of cholecystokinin by the duodenum when food enters.

78 They synthesize pancreatic juice.

79 These are alpha (secrete glucagon), beta (secrete insulin), and delta (secrete somatostatin).

80 They leave via fenestrated capillaries into the bloodstream. Fenestrations enable secretion.

Chapters 30 and 31: Respiratory system

81 Ciliated columnar, goblet, and basal cells.

82 Hyaline cartilage.

83 Surfactant is a phospholipoprotein. It is made by type II alveolar cells, and is found in the alveoli.

84 About 0.5 μm.

85 In Fig. I, arrow A is pointing towards a neutrophil, and B is pointing towards the alveolar wall. The alveoli are full of mucus and white blood cells, suggesting that an infection is present in the lung (e.g., pneumonia).

Chapters 32–34: Urinary system

86 The cortex.

87 It monitors the salt content of blood and can alter renin secretion, which results in the alteration of blood pressure, for example.

88 A simple cuboidal epithelium with microvilli.

89 A transitional epithelium.

90 In the image shown, the glomerulus looks highly abnormal, with very few capillaries, or mesangial cells, and there appears to be some sort of deposit in or between the cells in this structure. This is an example of kidney amyloidosis. It can be produced when plasma cells produce abnormal antibody fragments. These aggregate to form amyloid deposits, which block the glomeruli and prevent the kidney from working normally. A symptom might be protein in the urine.

Chapters 35 and 36: Female reproductive system

91 Oogenesis, and manufacture and secretion of hormones.

92 Epithelial tissue.

93 The follicular cells.

94 In Fig. K, arrow A is pointing towards a cluster of cells that look like cells from the sebaceous gland in the skin,

and B is pointing towards tissue similar to the epithelium in the skin. Both of these structures are not normally present in the ovary. This image is of an ovarian teratoma. This type of tumor develops from the germ cells in the ovary, and can result in cell types from ectodermal, mesodermal, and endodermal layers all appearing in the tumor. These types of tumor are 'encapsulated' and as such are normally benign.

95 A prepubescent girl would have many primordial follicles in the ovary, but no maturing oocytes. In a pregnant woman, much of the ovary would be taken up by a corpus luteum.

96 A secretion rich in glycogen.

97 This is because this region of the genital tract is likely to be invaded by foreign bacteria/organisms.

98 Colostrum is produced by the mammary glands in women in the first few days after the baby is born.

Chapters 37–39: Male reproductive system

99 Meiosis, to generate haploid cells.

100 The epididymis, vas deferens, ejaculatory duct, and urethra.

101 Prostate gland and seminal vesicles.

102 Through the rete testis indo the ductus efferentes and into the epididymis.

103 They secrete testosterone.

104 It is pseudostratified.

105 They are exocrine glands.

Chapters 40 and 41: Endocrine glands

106 Glands are formed from epithelia.

107 Hormones.

108 Colloid is reabsorbed from the lumen by the epithelial cells, and colloid is broken down with hydrolytic enzymes (in lysosomes) and then the active hormone secreted into the bloodstream.

109 This region secretes glucocorticoids, a type of steroid hormone, manufactured from lipid, hence the high level of lipid droplets.

Chapters 42 and 43: Lymphatic system

110 Peyer's patches.

111 Partially encapsulated lymphoid tissue.

112 The hilum.

113 In the thymus.

114 In the image shown (Fig. L), the mucosal lining of the appendix is enlarged compared to a normal appendix. This could be a sign of acute appendicitis, which could be investigated further by looking at higher magnification. Acute appendicitis results in a lack of blood supply (ischemia) followed by necrosis, bacteria can leak out into the lumen, which then fills with pus. Untreated, this can lead to septicemia.

Chapter 44: Eye and ear

115 The ciliary body is an outgrowth from the sclera that contains smooth muscle, which controls the shape of the lens.

116 The cornea is a specialized form of epithelium.

117 Ganglion cells.

118 In the lens.

119 It contains perilymph.

120 Phalangeal cells provide support for the hair cells, which sit in an apical cuticular plate formed by the phalangeal cells. The phalangeal cells are connected to the basilar membrane.

Index

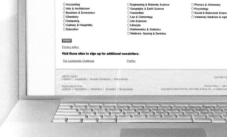
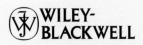

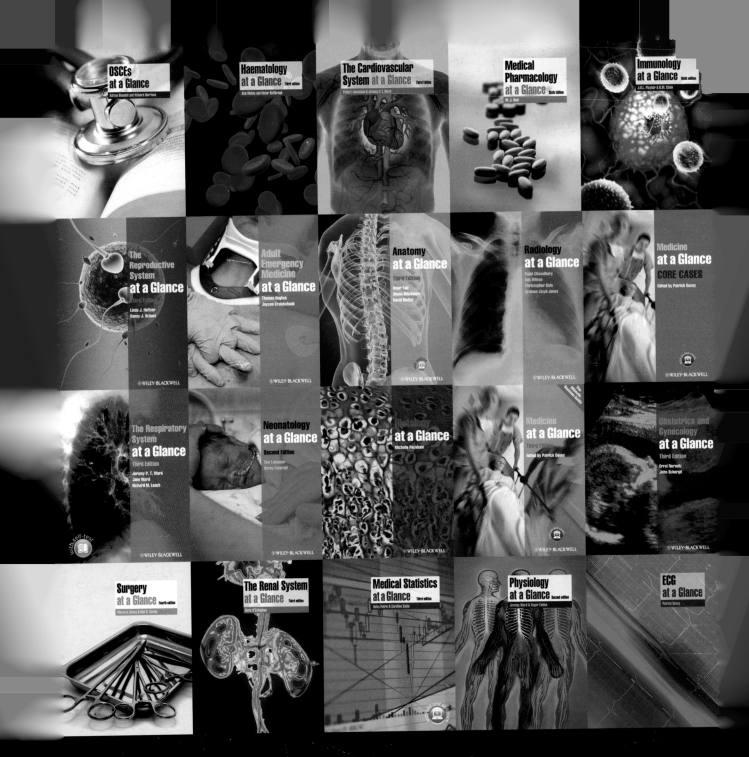

The at a Glance series

Popular double-page spread format • Coverage of core knowledge
Full-colour throughout • Self-assessment to test your knowledge • Expert authors

www.wileymedicaleducation.com

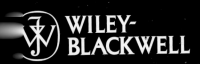